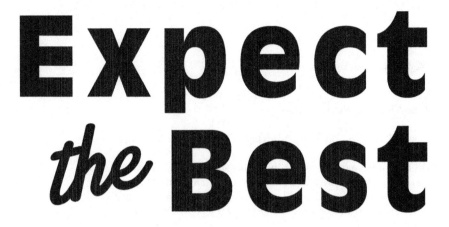

Expect *the* Best

YOUR GUIDE TO HEALTHY EATING BEFORE, DURING, AND AFTER PREGNANCY

Elizabeth M. Ward, MS, RD

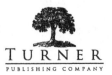

TURNER
PUBLISHING COMPANY

Turner Publishing Company
Nashville, Tennessee
New York, New York
www.turnerpublishing.com

Expect the Best, Revised Edition

The information contained in this book is based upon the research and personal and
professional experiences of the author. It is not intended as a substitute for consulting
with your physician or other healthcare provider. Any attempt to diagnose and treat an
illness should be done under the direction of a healthcare professional.

The publisher does not advocate the use of any particular healthcare protocol but
believes the information in this book should be available to the public. The publisher
and author are not responsible for any adverse effects or consequences resulting from
the use of the suggestions, preparations, or procedures discussed in this book. Should
the reader have any questions concerning the appropriateness of any procedures or
preparation mentioned, the author and the publisher strongly suggest consulting a professional healthcare advisor.

Interior design: Gary A. Rosenberg
Cover design: Maddie Cothren

Library of Congress Cataloging-in-Publication Data

Names: Ward, Elizabeth M., author. | Academy of Nutrition and Dietetics.
Title: Expect the best / Elizabeth M. Ward & the Academy of Nutrition and
  Dietetics.
Description: Revised edition. | Nashville, Tennessee : Turner Publishing,
  [2017] | Includes bibliographical references.
Identifiers: LCCN 2016050533 | ISBN 9781681626246 (pbk. : alk. paper)
Subjects: LCSH: Pregnancy--Nutritional aspects. | Mothers--Nutrition. |
  Exercise for pregnant women.
Classification: LCC RG559 .W36 2017 | DDC 618.2/4--dc23
LC record available at https://lccn.loc.gov/2016050533

Printed in the United States of America

10   9   8   7   6   5   4   3   2   1

Contents

Foreword

As a pediatrician, mom, and former director of a newborn nursery, I feel a special fondness for new and expectant moms and newborn babies. That's why I'm thrilled to be able to recommend the second edition of *Expect the Best,* by Elizabeth Ward, featuring the expertise of the Academy of Nutrition and Dietetics, our nation's leading group of nutrition professionals.

The journey into parenthood is one of the best times in life to focus on nutrition, for both yourself and your baby. The months and years before pregnancy offer the opportunity to quit vices such as smoking cigarettes, and to improve your diet in small ways that can make a big difference. It's challenging to make lifestyle changes, but it may be easier to try to improve knowing that good habits before and during pregnancy can affect both you and your child in a positive way long after he or she is born.

Filled with recommendations and information on a wide range of topics—including calories and weight gain, vitamins and minerals, exercise before, during, and after delivery, food safety, and the importance of healthy habits for expectant dads—this edition also features more than 60 easy, healthy recipes (nearly 40 of which are new) for time-crunched parents and parents-to-be. Above all, *Expect the Best* is informative, non-judgmental, and realistic, providing up-to-date knowledge to help you and your growing family start on your healthful journey and to stay on track when life gets busy.

I wish you the *best* as you put your *best* pregnancy foot forward and give your child the *best* start in life with the help of this new edition of *Expect the Best!*

—Jennifer Shu, MD, FAAP
Pediatrician and coauthor of
Heading Home with Your Newborn and *Food Fights*

Acknowledgments

For me, writing a book is kind of like having a baby. I remember only the good parts and forget any discomforts, which is why I am able to do it again!

This is my second time around with *Expect the Best*. You would think that writing another edition of your own book would be a breeze, and, in some respects it was. I love the subject matter, and I could talk about it all day. But the author in me fretted as much as any parent over the details, because I wanted to deliver the most complete, current, and interesting pregnancy nutrition book.

Fortunately, I had a lot of help. *Expect the Best* has the backing of the Academy of Nutrition and Dietetics, the world's largest organization of food and nutrition professionals. The Academy counts many experienced pregnancy and breastfeeding experts among their ranks of more than one hundred thousand credentialed practitioners. I am grateful that five registered dietitian nutritionists agreed to review drafts of *Expect the Best,* which made it a better resource for parents, and for those thinking about having a baby. I know that the reviewers took the utmost care to insure the accuracy of the information and to make it enjoyable for you to read. Thank you to Petra Lusche, MA, RDN/LD, IBCLC, CPT; Kim

Upton, RD; Hillary Wright, MEd, RD, LDN; Kathleen Zelman, MPH, RD; and one anonymous reviewer. You know who you are!

A big thank you goes out to the moms who spoke with me about their pregnancies. Their wisdom and perspective bring to life the advice that's doled out in *Expect the Best*. These seasoned parents offer tips and advice that you'll find useful and, at times, even humorous.

Writing a book is a group effort, and *Expect the Best* version 2.0 wouldn't have been possible without the expert editing, gentle guidance, and endless patience of Betsy Hornick, MS, RDN, and Allison Watzman at the Academy. I can't thank you enough for your expertise.

And last, but never least, I'd like to acknowledge my husband and children, who supported me on yet another book-writing adventure that made for long days in the office. I am also grateful to my family for sampling all the new recipes in *Expect the Best* and for offering tips to improve them so that you and your family can enjoy the book to its fullest.

Introduction

Maybe this is your first pregnancy, and having a baby is new to you. Perhaps you're an experienced parent, but you haven't had a child in a few years, and you're wondering what's new about the best way to eat before and during pregnancy. You could be breastfeeding an infant and thinking of having another baby in the near future. No matter what your situation, you're in the right place!

Clearly, you take great interest in doing your best as a parent or parent-to-be. You're reading this book, so you must be considering taking steps to help yourself and your child to a healthier future. When you have children, you want to do everything the "right" way. As the mother of three, I feel the same! It's easy to get confused by what you hear and read about healthy habits when you're preparing for pregnancy, or when you're pregnant or breastfeeding. It's comforting to know that following a balanced eating plan, along with engaging in other positive behaviors, can support your baby's well-being at birth and for years to come.

This is an exciting time to be having children because there is more information than ever about how you—and your partner—can have the healthiest baby possible. For example, we now know that fathers play a role in their future babies' health, and maybe not just in the way that you think. Men who assume that their contribution to making a baby begins and ends at conception should think again, as research suggests that a dad's health habits before his partner's pregnancy influence his child even more than was previously believed. Having a child is more of a partnership than it appears!

Medical advances have made it possible for many couples to work through fertility problems and go on to have successful pregnancies, and research suggests that lifestyle habits may affect your chances of conceiving through assisted reproductive techniques such as IVF. Women are delivering healthy babies well after age thirty-five, and eating right and getting regular physical activity help older moms' pregnancies progress more smoothly. In fact, moms of all ages benefit from a healthy eating plan and the suggested amount of exercise—whether they are carrying one child, twins, or more.

GET PRIMED FOR PREGNANCY

It used to be that women waited for a positive pregnancy test to quit smoking, stop drinking alcohol, and improve their food choices. Not anymore. Taking care of yourself before conception encourages fertility and reduces problems during pregnancy. Ideally, you should work with your doctor, nurse practitioner, or certified nurse-midwife, as well as with a registered dietitian nutritionist (RDN), to adopt habits that help you manage health issues (for example, iron-deficiency anemia) for months or even years ahead of having a child.

The sooner you start working on your health, the better. About half of the pregnancies in the United States are unexpected, so it pays to be prepared for pregnancy. A balanced diet prior to pregnancy helps ensure that your body has certain nutrients, such as iron, available to your baby after you've conceived, and it's important for your good health, too. If your diet wasn't so great before you got pregnant, that's OK. Just take it from here, eating what you need for the stage you're in now.

Once you're pregnant, you become your child's sole source of nourishment. That sounds like a lot of responsibility, but it's also exciting! Understanding how the environment in the womb influences lifelong well-being is a growing area of medical research that keeps turning up new discoveries. The notion that a mother can "program" her child's health with what she eats, and with other lifestyle habits, may seem far-fetched, but it's not. Of course, you don't have complete control over your child's development, but along with other healthy habits, adopting an eating plan built around nutrient-rich foods helps you sustain and replenish your nutrient reserves so that you and your baby thrive.

YOUR GUIDE TO A HEALTHIER PREGNANCY

Even if you're already eating well and you're physically active, the second edition of *Expect the Best* has plenty to offer you. Almost everything you need to know about a healthy lifestyle before, during, and after pregnancy is included in these pages, and it's not limited to food and nutrition.

This latest version of *Expect the Best* takes the most recent research and recommendations about pregnancy and breastfeeding from the country's top health organizations and translates them into easy-to-understand strategies for real life. The book explains in detail the Dietary Guidelines for Americans and MyPlate, a tool that serves up simple eating advice that will be useful for years to come. And *Expect the Best* emphasizes the best health habits to get ready to conceive a child.

More than 60 simple, nutritious, and delicious recipes in chapter 8 help you to live by experts' eating advice, and you'll see many recipes highlighted throughout the book as especially useful. In addition, real moms offer their tips and stories about pregnancy and breastfeeding experiences to help you better navigate this time of your life.

Here's a preview of what's ahead:

- The importance of achieving and maintaining a healthy weight before pregnancy, how much weight to gain when expecting and why, and postpregnancy weight-loss guidelines

- How much exercise you need in every stage of your life and every trimester, who should not work out during pregnancy, and what activities to avoid

- How diet and lifestyle affect your chances of conceiving a child

- What your male partner needs to do to increase his chances of fathering the healthiest child possible

- The nutrients necessary for your and your baby's well-being, before, during, and after pregnancy, why they matter, how much of them you need, and how to work them into an easy-to-follow eating plan that fits your lifestyle

- Realistic, balanced eating plans, whether you're thinking about having a baby, you're pregnant, or you're breastfeeding, and whether you want to gain weight, lose some pounds, or stay the same weight to prepare for motherhood

- How diet and lifestyle help you to dodge or manage the complications and discomforts of pregnancy

- Information about your diet and exercise during the "fourth trimester," the months immediately after delivering your child

- Food safety information to keep you healthy

- Dozens of resources on a range of topics, including childbirth, breastfeeding, infertility, and food safety

The information between these covers has been carefully reviewed for accuracy, and is backed by the Academy of Nutrition and Dietetics, the country's leading group of nutrition experts.

Ultimately, you'll make up your own mind about what to eat before and during pregnancy and after delivery. *Expect the Best* will be there to inspire—and gently guide—you on your journey with reliable and realistic information.

1

Prepregnancy: Starting from a Healthy Place

There's no need to wait for a positive pregnancy test to start working on a healthier lifestyle—you can begin today! When a balanced eating pattern, regular physical activity, and other healthy habits are part of your routine, your future child is more likely to benefit at birth and for a lifetime, and so are you. Now is a good time for you and your partner to think about how best to prepare for pregnancy.

MAKE A PERSONAL PLAN FOR A HEALTHIER PREGNANCY

You may think of preparing for pregnancy as little more than a single visit to your health care provider (internist, gynecologist, certified nurse-midwife, or nurse practitioner) in the months before trying for a baby, but experts see preconception health differently. The Centers for Disease Control and Prevention's (CDC's) Preconception Health and Health Care Initiative focuses on steps you can take before conception to optimize your health, which in turn will help nourish and protect your future baby, whether or not this is your first child.

Preconception wellness is about getting healthy and staying that way. You may be surprised to learn that preconception health is important for men as well as women. Why is your well-being, and that of your partner, so essential before conception occurs? While there are no guarantees, being in the best health possible when you conceive a child reduces his or her chances of being born early (preterm), of having a low birth weight (under five pounds, eight ounces) or a high birth weight (more than eight pounds, thirteen ounces), and of being affected by birth defects or other problems. It also makes it easier to return to your prepregnancy weight.

Living the healthiest lifestyle you can and controlling medical conditions to the best of your ability gives your child a head start in life. Preconception health is especially important when you consider that half of all pregnancies in the United States are unplanned or unexpected. The risk for birth defects and other problems is greatest during the first ten weeks of pregnancy, also known as the embryo stage. During this time, women may not realize they are expecting, and most have not yet seen a health care professional to learn about what to avoid and what to include in their diets.

Make your prebaby health, and your well-being between pregnancies, a high priority. If your primary care provider (the doctor or nurse practitioner you see for annual physicals and when you are ill) doesn't bring up your preconception plan, the CDC suggests that you start this important conversation. There's no official age to begin planning for a child, but it's reasonable to start taking your good health seriously by age eighteen, or even earlier. You can begin the discussion about preconception care with your primary health care provider, your registered dietitian nutritionist (RDN), and even your dentist by letting them know that you're planning for a child, whether it's sooner or later.

Preconception care should be ongoing and personalized for conditions such as being overweight or underweight, disordered eating, celiac disease, high blood pressure, prediabetes and diabetes, polycystic ovary syndrome (PCOS), or a combination of issues. If you've ever delivered a low-birth-weight baby, a preterm infant (a child born before thirty-seven weeks of pregnancy), or a child with a birth defect, or if you've had a pregnancy end in infant death, always seek medical advice before trying to conceive. If you're experiencing infertility, consider seeing a specialist.

The next two sections of this chapter consist of preconception checklists for mom and dad.

A PRECONCEPTION TO-DO LIST FOR MOMS-TO-BE

In addition to undergoing regular medical checkups and a thorough physical examination before conception, future moms can take several steps to improve their wellness.

✓ Check Your Weight

You're trying for a baby, and you may have heard that having a body weight within the healthy range could make it easier to get pregnant. That's because either too much or too little body fat interferes with a woman's ability to conceive, both naturally and by using methods such as in vitro fertilization (IVF). Research also suggests that excess body fat interferes with a man's fertility. If both you and your partner are overweight, it could take longer to conceive than if only one of you needs to shed some pounds.

In addition to influencing fertility, being obese (having a BMI of 29.9 or above) at the time of conception may increase the chances for having a child with structural defects, including those of the neural tube, heart, and limbs. Defects of the neural tube, which forms your baby's brain and spinal column, are the most likely structural birth defect in children born to obese women. Spina bifida is the most common kind of neural tube defect (NTD). Consuming adequate folic acid early in pregnancy helps reduce the risk for spina bifida in many women. Nevertheless, even adequate folic acid consumption might not protect obese women from having a pregnancy affected by an NTD.

Starting pregnancy at a healthy weight (a BMI of 18.5 to 24.9) gives your child a better chance of developing normally and supports your health by helping to reduce the risk of the following problems:

- High blood pressure in mom during pregnancy
- Gestational diabetes (diabetes during pregnancy) in mom, and low blood glucose levels in baby at birth
- Induced labor (which can require more medication and lead to a longer labor)
- A larger baby, making him or her more difficult to deliver and increasing the chances for cesarean delivery
- A child who is at a greater risk for becoming overweight during childhood and beyond
- Preterm (before thirty-seven weeks) labor and delivery
- A pregnancy that ends in stillbirth (death in the womb after the twentieth week of pregnancy)
- Shorter time spent breastfeeding

REALITY CHECK: BODY WEIGHT DOESN'T DETERMINE DESTINY

There's plenty of doom and gloom about body weight before pregnancy. Sure, there are downsides to being underweight and overweight before and during pregnancy. The good news is that you and your partner can start eating better and exercising more right now to get you to a healthier place before pregnancy. If you're already pregnant, it's possible to have a healthy pregnancy even when your weight at conception wasn't within the healthy range. There's more information about nutrition and weight gain during pregnancy in chapter 4.

How will you know what body weight is right for you before trying for a baby? There's no single weight that's best. Rather, there is a range. With the exception of very muscular and short-statured people, determining one's BMI is the most accurate way for nearly everyone to know what range their body weight falls into. BMI indicates body fat based on a (nonpregnant) adult's height and weight. Measure your height without shoes. For the greatest accuracy, weigh yourself naked, first thing in the morning, after using the bathroom and before eating or drinking. Then consult the BMI chart on pages 10–11 to determine your BMI.

You can also find your BMI with the BMI calculator from the National Heart, Lung, and Blood Institute (NHLBI) at www.nhlbisupport.com/bmi.

Getting information about your BMI is a great first step to understanding what, if any, action you may need to take regarding your body weight. Talk with your doctor, nurse practitioner, or registered dietitian nutritionist (RDN) about your BMI and whether it's best to lose weight, put on some pounds, or stay at the same weight. No matter what your goal, you'll need a balanced food plan. See chapter 3 for more information about balanced eating.

✓ Bridge the Nutrient Gaps in Your Diet

You may look and feel great, but if you're like many Americans, you could be short on nutrients that would help you stay in tip-top shape while you are trying to conceive, even if your weight is in the healthy range.

The 2015–2020 Dietary Guidelines for Americans (Dietary Guidelines or DGA), a joint effort of the US Department of Agriculture and the US Department of Health and Human Services, serves as the blueprint for healthy eating and exercise for Americans over the age of two. According to the Dietary Guidelines, adults often fail to include enough of the following nutrients in their eating plans on a regular basis:

- Fiber
- Calcium
- Potassium
- Vitamin D

In addition, the guidelines recommend that women should include adequate amounts of the following two nutrients during their childbearing years:

- Iron
- Folic acid

Research suggests that many of us may have lower than suggested intakes for additional nutrients, including vitamins A, C, E, and K, choline, and the mineral magnesium. Generally speaking, adults and children don't meet their needs for many of these nutrients because they don't eat enough whole grains, fruits, vegetables, and dairy foods on a regular basis.

Food is best for getting the nutrients you need before, during, and after pregnancy. But although a multivitamin/mineral pill is no match for a balanced diet, it is beneficial for many women in their childbearing years. Your eating plan could easily fall short for several vitamins and minerals if you:

- eat a low-calorie diet or are currently dieting;

BODY MASS INDEX																	
	Normal						Overweight					Obese					
BMI	19	20	21	22	23	24	25	26	27	28	29	30	31	32	33	34	35
Height (inches)	Body Weight (pounds)																
58	91	96	100	105	110	115	119	124	129	134	138	143	148	153	158	162	167
59	94	99	104	109	114	119	124	128	133	138	143	148	153	158	163	168	173
60	97	102	107	112	118	123	128	133	138	143	148	153	158	163	168	174	179
61	100	106	111	116	122	127	132	137	143	148	153	158	164	169	174	180	185
62	104	109	115	120	126	131	136	142	147	153	158	164	169	175	180	186	191
63	107	113	118	124	130	135	141	146	152	158	163	169	175	180	186	191	197
64	110	116	122	128	134	140	145	151	157	163	169	174	180	186	192	197	204
65	114	120	126	132	138	144	150	156	162	168	174	180	186	192	198	204	210
66	118	124	130	136	142	148	155	161	167	173	179	186	192	198	204	210	216
67	121	127	134	140	146	153	159	166	172	178	185	191	198	204	211	217	223
68	125	131	138	144	151	158	164	171	177	184	190	197	203	210	216	223	230
69	128	135	142	149	155	162	169	176	182	189	196	203	209	216	223	230	236
70	132	139	146	153	160	167	174	181	188	195	202	209	216	222	229	236	243
71	136	143	150	157	165	172	179	186	193	200	208	215	222	229	236	243	250
72	140	147	154	162	169	177	184	191	199	206	213	221	228	235	242	250	258
73	144	151	159	166	174	182	189	197	204	212	219	227	235	242	250	257	265
74	148	155	163	171	179	186	194	202	210	218	225	233	241	249	256	264	272
75	152	160	168	176	184	192	200	208	216	224	232	240	248	256	264	272	279
76	156	164	172	180	189	197	205	213	221	230	238	246	254	263	271	279	287

- are overweight;

- have had weight-loss surgery;

- have a condition (e.g., celiac disease) that reduces the body's absorption of vitamins A, D, E, and K;

- smoke cigarettes;

- avoid or restrict foods from any food group;

BODY MASS INDEX																		
Obese				Extreme Obesity														
36	37	38	39	40	41	42	43	44	45	46	47	48	49	50	51	52	53	54
Body Weight (pounds)																		
172	177	181	186	191	196	201	205	210	215	220	224	229	234	239	244	248	253	258
178	183	188	193	198	203	208	212	217	222	227	232	237	242	247	252	257	262	267
184	189	194	199	204	209	215	220	225	230	235	240	245	250	255	261	266	271	276
190	195	201	206	211	217	222	227	232	238	243	248	254	259	264	269	275	280	285
196	202	207	213	218	224	229	235	240	246	251	256	262	267	273	278	284	289	295
203	208	214	220	225	231	237	242	248	254	259	265	270	278	282	287	293	299	304
209	215	221	227	232	238	244	250	256	262	267	273	279	285	291	296	302	308	314
216	222	228	234	240	246	252	258	264	270	276	282	288	294	300	306	312	318	324
223	229	235	241	247	253	260	266	272	278	284	291	297	303	309	315	322	328	334
230	236	242	249	255	261	268	274	280	287	293	299	306	312	319	325	331	338	344
236	243	249	256	262	269	276	282	289	295	302	308	315	322	328	335	341	348	354
243	250	257	263	270	277	284	291	297	304	311	318	324	331	338	345	351	358	365
250	257	264	271	278	285	292	299	306	313	320	327	334	341	348	355	362	369	376
257	265	272	279	286	293	301	308	315	322	329	338	343	351	358	365	372	379	386
265	272	279	287	294	302	309	316	324	331	338	346	353	361	368	375	383	390	397
272	280	288	295	302	310	318	325	333	340	348	355	363	371	378	386	393	401	408
280	287	295	303	311	319	326	334	342	350	358	365	373	381	389	396	404	412	420
287	295	303	311	319	327	335	343	351	359	367	375	383	391	399	407	415	423	431
295	304	312	320	328	336	344	353	361	369	377	385	394	402	410	418	426	435	443

- eat a gluten-free diet;

- take medications that interfere with the absorption and/or metabolism of certain micronutrients, including proton pump inhibitors (PPI) for reflux disease, or metformin to control blood glucose levels;

- don't adhere to the eating patterns suggested by MyPlate (see chapter 3).

FOCUS ON FOLATE

Folate (and its synthetic cousin, folic acid) is mentioned in the 2015–2020 DGA as a nutrient worthy of attention during the childbearing years. Women whose diets fall short of fruits, vegetables, legumes (beans), and enriched grains, and who do not take dietary supplements, might not consume the recommended amount of folate every day. Folate and folic acid help to prevent neural tube defects within the first month of pregnancy, when the neural tube forms. The neural tube eventually develops into your baby's spine and brain. According to the US Public Health Service, women who have had a pregnancy affected by a neural tube defect may be advised to consume 4 milligrams (mg) of folic acid every day for one month prior to conceiving and for the first three months of pregnancy. That's ten times the regular recommended amount of 4 micrograms (mcg). You may require additional folic acid if you're pregnant with more than one child, or if you have diabetes or epilepsy. Discuss your folic acid needs with your health care provider. Read up on folic acid and folate in chapter 2.

Multivitamin/mineral supplements help to fill gaps for essential nutrients in your eating plan. However, many dietary supplements are just what their name implies, supplements, and no single supplement or combination of supplements can duplicate the mix of nutrients and other substances in food that work together to offer health benefits. Nor can dietary supplements fix a poor eating plan. For example, most supplements are missing appreciable amounts of several of the nutrients identified in the Dietary Guidelines as being deficient in the diet, including potassium and calcium. And multivitamin/mineral supplements do not contain the carbohydrate, protein, and fat required to produce the energy that fuels everything that happens in your body. Nevertheless, taking a multivitamin/mineral supplement is a low-risk, relatively low-cost approach to improving the chances of having the healthiest baby possible.

Several studies show that taking a multivitamin containing at least 400 mcg of folic acid before pregnancy reduces the likelihood of congenital (present at birth) defects, including those affecting the neural tube, heart, limbs, and palate. Taking a multivitamin on a regular basis before pregnancy may lower the chances of having a baby who's small for gestational age (a baby smaller than the usual size for the number of weeks of pregnancy) and the chances of preterm birth in women with a body weight in the healthy range. Research suggests that women who take multivitamins daily before and during early pregnancy have a 55 percent lower risk of miscarriage than women who take no multivitamins. Preliminary evidence also suggests that a daily multivitamin with folic acid and iron may reduce the risk of autism spectrum disorders (ASD) and developmental disabilities, particularly in women with inefficient folate metabolism, which is a genetic trait. It's not possible to know if you process folate inefficiently without a specific blood test, although the condition is relatively rare. If you're concerned, speak with your doctor about the test.

When you become pregnant, your health care provider may recommend a prenatal multivitamin with higher levels of nutrients, including folic acid and iron, instead of regular multivitamins. Do not take both types of pills at the same time. With the exception of calcium, and possibly vitamin D, it may be unnecessary to take individual supplements when taking a prenatal vitamin. Discuss your individual nutrient needs with your doctor, nurse practitioner, or RDN.

> **Words of Motherly Wisdom**
>
> "As soon as we decided to have a baby, I started taking a multivitamin every day. My husband did, too. I've taken vitamins ever since."
> —Sarah

FINDING THE RIGHT MULTIVITAMIN

There are many types of multivitamin pills to choose from. Look for the following qualities when making your choice:

About 100 percent of the Daily Value (DV) of the nutrients contained in the pill, including iron, folic acid, and iodine (but not vitamin A). Since you're also eating, you will get nutrients from food, so there's no need to overdo it with supplements. The DVs are recommended intakes for adults who are neither pregnant nor nursing, and they are a useful guide for women trying to conceive.

Fewer than 3,000 international units (IU) of vitamin A (1,500 micrograms), with the majority of it in the form of beta-carotene. Consuming excessive amounts of vitamin A as retinol (the preformed variety that is often found in dietary supplements and is called *vitamin A acetate* or *palmitate*) increases the chances for birth defects in a developing baby. In addition, too much vitamin A from retinol is toxic to the liver and bad for your bones. Beta-carotene, the raw material that the body converts to vitamin A, is safer. Supplemental beta-carotene is not known to increase the risk of birth defects.

No extras. Skip supplements that contain herbs and other botanicals, as well as extra ingredients such as amino acids and caffeine. They add to the cost of multivitamins, and many have not been proven safe for pregnant women.

✓ Get a Medical Checkup

It's important to know if you have certain health conditions, such as low iron or high blood glucose levels, before you get pregnant. Taking control of medical conditions prior to pregnancy will help you, and your baby, once you're expecting. Regular screening, such as a yearly blood test (often referred to as a complete blood count, or CBC) may turn up issues that you can attend to well before pregnancy.

Dietary iron, found in fortified grains, meat, poultry, and seafood, helps you to maintain proper levels of iron in your body. You have iron circulating in your blood to meet your immediate needs, and your body stores iron, too. Several studies suggest that the amount of iron stored in your body at the time of conception is linked to your chances for iron-deficiency anemia later in pregnancy, when iron needs increase. Iron-deficiency anemia during pregnancy raises the risk of having a preterm delivery and a low-birth-weight baby.

You may be one of the millions of women of childbearing age with an iron deficiency that causes anemia, and you might not even know it. For example, you may accept the fatigue linked to iron-deficiency anemia as part of your busy life, so you overlook it as a sign of the condition. It's harder to replenish depleted iron stores once pregnancy has begun, so it's best to get the iron you need before you conceive. It's harder, but possible, to deal with an iron deficiency when you're pregnant because your body demands even more iron during pregnancy.

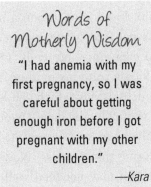

Words of Motherly Wisdom

"I had anemia with my first pregnancy, so I was careful about getting enough iron before I got pregnant with my other children."

—*Kara*

Ask your health care provider to test your blood for ferritin, a good indicator of the amount of iron you have for later use. Along with other blood tests, a low ferritin level in the bloodstream means you have iron deficiency and probably need to take iron supplements before you conceive to help ensure that your body is storing enough iron. It may take several months of eating a more iron-rich diet and taking iron supplements to correct iron-deficiency anemia.

✓ Deal with Prediabetes and Diabetes

Experts estimate that one in three Americans, including women in their childbearing years, has prediabetes. Prediabetes is a blood glucose level that registers outside the normal range but is not elevated enough for a diagnosis of diabetes. Having elevated blood glucose before pregnancy may mean a greater chance of developing gestational diabetes (diabetes during pregnancy) and of developing type 2 diabetes after delivery.

There are several possible consequences of prediabetes and type 2 diabetes when you're expecting. During pregnancy, extra glucose in your blood can cause your baby to grow too large. Women with prediabetes and diabetes during pregnancy may require a cesarean delivery because of the baby's size. Larger babies at birth may become overweight as children and are at higher risk for developing type 2 diabetes later in life. In addition, when a baby is "fed" extra glucose during pregnancy, its pancreas produces excess insulin, the hormone that helps glucose to gain entry into cells. Once born, a baby no longer receives surplus glucose from his mother. Yet the baby's body continues to produce too much insulin, which can lead to low blood glucose levels in a newborn. Eventually, the baby's pancreas stops making excess insulin, which may take hours or days and he or she may require treatment in the hospital during that process. Newborns with low blood glucose levels for any reason may not feed well, may have breathing problems, and may be irritable or listless.

Jaundice is another possible complication that is more common in babies delivered by women with diabetes. Jaundice is the yellowing of skin caused by a buildup of old red blood cells that the body should be disposing. Babies with jaundice are also more likely to have low supplies of iron in their livers, which can result in iron-deficiency anemia.

It's possible to have prediabetes and not know it because the condition is often symptom-free. Measuring your glucose level as part of a blood test after fasting is a good way to find out if you're at risk. (A fasting level is obtained after going nine hours without eating.) A normal fasting blood glucose value when you're not pregnant is below 100 milligrams per deciliter (mg/dl). If you have prediabetes, your fasting blood glucose level will measure between 100 and 125 mg/dl. When a person's fasting blood glucose level rises to 126 mg/dl or above, that's diabetes.

The older you get, the greater your risk for prediabetes, but it's possible to have it in your twenties and thirties. The good news is that even when your blood glucose level is higher than normal, it is likely to drop when you lose weight, improve your eating habits, and exercise regularly. For example, for a person weighing two hundred pounds, losing just ten to fifteen pounds can slow or even reverse prediabetes.

IF YOU HAVE DIABETES, GET BLOOD GLUCOSE UNDER CONTROL

If you have diabetes, you've got company. According to the Centers for Disease Control and Prevention, thirteen million women over age twenty in the United States had diabetes (type 1 and type 2) as of 2012, a number that has likely increased by now. Women with either type of diabetes are three times more likely than women without diabetes to deliver a baby with a birth defect, to miscarry, or to have a pregnancy end in infant death. The infants of women who had diabetes throughout pregnancy are also prone to higher blood pressure and to becoming overweight in childhood.

Nevertheless, there is good news. Getting control of your glucose level greatly increases your chances of having a healthy baby. Before you try to get pregnant, the American Diabetes Association recommends that you have an A1C (also known as glycated hemoglobin) level as close to less than 7 percent as possible. Your A1C concentration reflects the average of your blood glucose levels for the past few months and provides a clearer picture of blood glucose control than any single blood glucose reading. It's important to strive for good blood glucose control at all times during your childbearing years since you might not know that you're expecting for several weeks after conception occurs, which is a critical time for a baby's development.

A fasting blood glucose level is typically part of the blood test in a complete physical examination, but ask for it anyway, especially if you are overweight and have any of the following risk factors for diabetes:

- High blood pressure

- Overweight or obesity

- Low levels of high-density lipoprotein cholesterol (HDL, the "good" cholesterol) and elevated triglycerides (fat) in the blood

- A family history of diabetes

- A history of gestational diabetes or giving birth to a baby weighing more than nine pounds

- Belonging to an ethnic group that is at high risk for diabetes: American Indians/Alaskan Natives, non-Hispanic Blacks, Hispanics, Asian Americans, and non-Hispanic Whites

✓ Check Your Thyroid Function

The thyroid gland, located in the lower front part of the neck, produces thyroxine, the hormone that controls the pace of many body functions, including metabolism. When the thyroid is sluggish, a condition called *hypothyroidism,* thyroxine levels fall. As a result, you might feel colder, tire more easily, have drier skin, become forgetful or depressed, and have bouts of constipation. In *hyperthyroidism,* excess thyroxine speeds up the metabolism, causing an array of symptoms such as irritability, increased heart rate, anxiety, weight loss in spite of a good appetite, and irregular menstrual periods.

Hypothyroidism is one of the most common thyroid disorders. It is more prevalent in women than in men, and it's particularly common in women in their childbearing years. Health experts don't agree that all pregnant women should be screened for hypothyroidism during pregnancy, but it doesn't hurt to have your thyroid function checked before you conceive and when you become pregnant, especially for women at high risk for thyroid disease, such as those who have previously been treated for hyperthyroidism or who have a positive family history of thyroid disease. Testing thyroid function is important in these groups because hypothyroidism can be symptom-free.

> ### Words of Motherly Wisdom
>
> "I was more tired than I had ever been, even when I got enough sleep, and I had a hard time remembering things at work and at home. My doctor ordered a blood test, and I found out my thyroid function was low. Now I take medication for it, and I feel great!"
>
> —Peg

By the end of the first trimester, your child's thyroid will be making its own thyroid hormones. Until then, the baby is dependent on you for the correct balance of thyroid hormones that help to maximize his brain development. A developing baby who has started to produce thyroid hormones also requires iodine, a mineral that your diet must supply, which serves as a raw material for making the thyroid hormones in your body and in baby's. See chapter 2 for more about iodine.

✓ Update Your Vaccinations

Women in their childbearing years should keep their vaccinations current, as should we all. Make sure you have had the following vaccines before conceiving:

- Tetanus, diphtheria, pertussis booster

- Measles, mumps, and rubella

- Varicella (chicken pox)

- Human papillomavirus (HPV) for women and men

- Meningococcus

- Hepatitis B

- Influenza (flu) vaccine (made from an inactivated virus)

- Pneumococcus

Discuss with your health care provider how long to wait to try for a baby after receiving any vaccine or booster shot.

FEELING BLUE?

Your emotional well-being is just as important as your physical health. If you have felt sad or hopeless lately, or if you derive little pleasure in life, you could be depressed. The US Preventive Services Task Force (USPSTF) recommends screening for depression in the general population, including pregnant women and those who have given birth. Mom's depression can affect her baby after delivery, too. Depressed mothers tend to be more withdrawn and do less to support a newborn's development. Talk with your health care provider about your feelings, and get the help you need.

✓ Visit Your Dentist

Your mouth can be an indicator of your overall health. Some studies suggest a link between the germs in the mouth that cause gum disease and having a preterm or low-birth-weight baby. It's best to try to take care of any necessary dental work, including cavities and gum disease, before getting pregnant. It's OK, and recommended, to get dental check-ups throughout pregnancy. Confirm that you are not pregnant before having dental X-rays and local anesthetic, both of which can be risky for a developing baby.

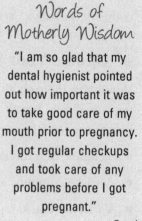

Words of Motherly Wisdom

"I am so glad that my dental hygienist pointed out how important it was to take good care of my mouth prior to pregnancy. I got regular checkups and took care of any problems before I got pregnant."

—Sarah

Here are some other dental hygiene tips for mothers-to-be:

- See your dentist immediately if you are having any dental problems, such as bleeding gums, whether you are pregnant or not.

- Brush after every meal, floss at least once a day, and use a fluoride rinse daily.

- If you're at risk for gum disease, have frequent dental visits. Discuss with your dentist how often you should be seen.

- To prevent tooth decay and gum disease, eat carbohydrate-rich foods, such as bread and crackers, along with other foods, such as meat, poultry, and seafood, and consume sweet desserts soon after meals, if at all. Consider eating cheese at the end of a meal instead of cookies, cake, or ice cream. Cheese neutralizes the mouth bacteria that can cause cavities, while sugars and other carbohydrates provide the energy the bacteria need to thrive.

- Consume enough calcium. The calcium in milk strengthens the bone in your jaw that helps to hold your teeth in place, and the vitamin D in fortified milk and other foods and in dietary supplements helps your body to better absorb calcium. If you don't drink milk, get calcium from other calcium-rich foods, including calcium-fortified orange juice and soy or almond milk. See more about calcium on page 78.

✓ Mind Your Medications

Many prescription and over-the-counter medications that you may take without a second thought could be dangerous to your unborn child, especially during the first trimester, when her organs are forming. That goes double for recreational drugs, including marijuana.

Because of the risk of miscarriage and birth defects, excessive levels of vitamin A in acne medications such as isotretinoin should be avoided by women who are pregnant or who may become pregnant. It is extremely important for sexually active women who could become pregnant and who take vitamin A–based acne medications to use an effective method of birth control. Women of childbearing age who take these medications are advised to undergo monthly pregnancy tests to make sure they are not pregnant.

Even seemingly harmless over-the-counter medications, such as common pain relievers, can be unsafe during pregnancy. This doesn't mean that all medications are off-limits during pregnancy, especially some used to treat chronic conditions. For example, women with an underactive thyroid must continue on thyroid medications throughout pregnancy to ensure proper neurological development in their child.

It's always a good idea to consider the risks and benefits of everything you take, including dietary supplements such as herbs and botanicals. You might think that because herbs and other dietary supplements are made from plants, they're OK, but that's not necessarily true, especially during pregnancy.

Unlike over-the-counter and prescription medications, dietary supplement products are not reviewed by the Food and Drug Administration (FDA) before they go on the market. (The FDA is responsible for taking action against any unsafe dietary supplement, however.) In addition, because herbs and botanicals are not regulated, you can't always be sure of what you are buying. That doesn't mean all herbs and botanicals are not worthy or useful. For example, ginger is considered acceptable for use during pregnancy, and it can be quite effective for treating nausea. Yet there is only limited scientific evidence that herbs and botanicals are safe during pregnancy and breastfeeding. Research suggests that the following are potentially dangerous for a woman who's expecting or nursing a child and should be avoided:

- Feverfew
- Mugwort
- Blue cohosh
- Goldenseal
- Juniper berry
- Chasteberry
- Rue
- Pennyroyal oil
- Ephedra

In addition, some herbal products, including guarana, yerba mate, kola nut, and green tea extract, may contain varying amounts of caffeine, which may influence your ability to conceive. (See page 53 for more on caffeine.) The FDA does not require that herbal products have a label saying how much caffeine they contain. When it comes to herbs and botanicals, until we know more about their safety, it's better to avoid most of them when you're trying to conceive or are pregnant or nursing. Speak with your health care professional and your pharmacist about what medications and dietary supplements are safe when you're trying to conceive, when you are pregnant, or when you're breastfeeding.

HERBAL TEA ALERT

Although herbal teas are caffeine-free, there simply isn't enough scientific evidence about the safety of many teas made from herbs and other plant parts, such as roots (with the exception of ginger). The chances are that the types of herbal teas in filtered bags that are available on supermarket shelves, such as chamomile and peppermint, are safe in reasonable amounts. For more information about herbal teas and dietary supplements, visit the website of the National Center for Complementary and Integrative Health at https://nccih.nih.gov/health/herbsataglance.htm.

✓ Assess Your Alcohol Intake

Health experts suggest avoiding alcohol at all times during pregnancy, but what about before? Experts such as the CDC and the March of Dimes advise that drinking alcohol and trying to conceive do not mix. Although moderate drinking—defined as no more than one drink a day for women—may be linked to certain health benefits depending on the type of drink, sipping two or more alcoholic beverages on a regular basis (known as heavy drinking) may make it more difficult to conceive a child and carry the pregnancy to term. Another reason to avoid beer, wine, and hard liquor when trying for a baby: you could become pregnant and not know it for several weeks. Drinking alcohol in pregnancy is linked to a greater risk for miscarriage, which is the loss of a pregnancy before twenty weeks. One large study of nearly ninety-three thousand Danish women found that those who drank one and a half drinks a week during the first trimester had one and a half times the risk of miscarriage (up to sixteen weeks of pregnancy) than those who drank no alcohol. An earlier study from the same country discovered that women who consumed five or more drinks a week during pregnancy were three times more likely to have a stillborn baby than women who had less than one drink a week.

Alcohol is a compound capable of causing birth defects. It passes easily and swiftly through the placenta—the organ that removes waste products and delivers oxygen and nutrients—to your child. The effects of alcohol can cause irreversible harm, particularly during the first trimester, when the baby's organs form at a rapid rate. Drinking alcohol on a regular basis in the first three months of pregnancy can cause abnormal facial features in your child, and your baby's brain can be harmed by exposure to alcohol at any time during your pregnancy. Binge drinking—defined for a woman as four or more drinks in a five-hour time span—is one of the riskiest patterns of alcohol intake when expecting a child.

REALITY CHECK:
IS ALCOHOL REALLY THAT BAD?

The definition of "a drink" might be smaller than you imagine. Experts consider a drink to be one of the following: 12 ounces of regular beer, 8 ounces of malt liquor, 5 ounces of wine, or $1^1/_2$ ounces of 80-proof distilled spirits (such as rum, vodka, or whiskey). If you had a drink or two before you realized you were pregnant, try not to worry. While there is no known safe level for alcohol intake during pregnancy, most of the evidence about alcohol's effects on babies comes from observing the results of heavy drinking in children after the fact. The effects of low and moderate drinking during pregnancy have not been well studied in humans, and for good reason. It's unreasonable to expect researchers to take chances with a baby's development by encouraging their moms to drink any amount of alcohol. Although there is a lack of evidence about the effects of lower alcohol consumption, discuss your concerns with your doctor, nurse-midwife, or nurse practitioner.

Heavy drinking during pregnancy increases the risk of mental retardation, learning disabilities, birth defects, and emotional and behavioral problems, such as those included in fetal alcohol syndrome (FAS). FAS is one of the worst consequences of drinking alcohol, and it's included as part of Fetal Alcohol Spectrum Disorders (FASD). FASD is a group of conditions that vary from mild to severe and include a broad array of physical defects and cognitive, behavioral, and emotional problems. In addition to increasing the risk for learning disabilities and birth defects, consuming alcohol during pregnancy also increases the risk of having a low-birth-weight baby. Low-birth-weight babies are prone to health problems at delivery and later on in life.

✓ Consider Caffeine Consumption

As anyone with a caffeine habit knows, caffeine is a stimulant that perks you up. For the first time ever, the 2015–2020 Dietary Guidelines for Americans addressed caffeine, concluding that up to 400 milligrams (mg) of caffeine daily can be part of a healthy eating pattern.

Most experts say that reasonable amounts of caffeine, considered to be less than 200 mg a day, probably have little effect on fertility, but that more might delay conception. (See page 55 for the caffeine content of common beverages and foods.) However, the evidence about caffeine and conception is murky because there aren't a lot of reliable studies on the subject. Women using assisted reproductive technology (ART) to help them get pregnant may want to take note of a study in the journal *Human Reproduction* that compared the caffeine habits of women with conception rates. Those who used in vitro fertilization (IVF) and consumed less than 50 mg of caffeine daily had higher conception rates than women using IVF who consumed more caffeine.

It never hurts to be cautious when trying to conceive, but it's good to know that you probably don't have to completely cut out caffeine. In fact, you may not need to make any changes at all. Coffee is the major source of caffeine in the United States, but caffeine can also be found in other beverages, certain foods, and certain medications. See chapter 2 to tally your daily caffeine intake and decide whether to cut down to possibly improve your fertility and your pregnancy.

FROM THE RECIPE FILE

You don't have to give up on coffee completely to cut back on caffeine consumption. Try the tasty recipe for Café Au Lait on page 222.

✓ Stop Smoking

Smoking before pregnancy jeopardizes your health by increasing your chances for lung and heart disease, among other problems. During pregnancy, smoking decreases your capacity to tolerate the demands that pregnancy will put on your body. Smoking can also make getting pregnant difficult. Studies show that women who smoke often have more trouble conceiving than nonsmokers and are more likely to miscarry.

Smoking during pregnancy is harmful for mother and child. Cigarette smoke contains thousands of dangerous chemicals in addition to nicotine. Although it's uncertain how many of these chemicals can hurt you and your baby, it's certain that nicotine and carbon monoxide interfere with your baby's supply of oxygen, which he must have to grow and develop properly. Smoking cigarettes during pregnancy increases the risk of having a smaller baby, having a preterm baby, stillbirth, and newborn death. Smoking also increases the risk of facial deformities, such as cleft lip or cleft palate.

If you're a smoker who is planning to quit once you're pregnant, don't wait. It's unwise to put off kicking the cigarette habit because it may take several tries to give it up for good. If you quit smoking but your partner does not, your baby's growth and birth weight can be affected by exposure to secondhand smoke during pregnancy. Women who are exposed to secondhand smoke may have more trouble getting pregnant, too. Encourage your partner and other people whom you live with or whom you are around a lot to quit smoking or at least not to smoke when you're present. You're more likely to stay off cigarettes when you get support from your friends and your family.

Don't plan on lighting up again once the baby is born. Babies who are exposed to secondhand smoke are more likely to suffer from lower-respiratory illnesses (such as bronchitis and pneumonia), asthma, and ear infections, and they run a greater risk of sudden infant death syndrome (SIDS).

You many think that e-cigarettes are safer than the regular kind, but it's not clear if that's true. E-cigarettes contain nicotine and other toxic compounds, and nobody knows the effects of repeated exposure to these substances on you and your developing baby.

✓ Move Around, and Often

You likely know the many benefits of exercise, and perhaps you're already active on most days of the week. Or maybe you're too tired or too busy to exercise regularly. But knowing how physical activity influences your health may help motivate you to move around more often. Here are some of the top benefits:

- Easier weight control

- Improved mood

- Better sleep

- Increased energy

- A stronger heart and a lower pulse rate

- Better muscle tone, more flexible joints, and stronger bones

- A reduced risk of type 2 diabetes, and better management of blood glucose levels in type 1 and type 2 diabetes

- Better blood pressure control

- Improved circulation

- Clearer thinking

Words of Motherly Wisdom

"Try not to get overwhelmed by having to exercise if you don't usually work out. I started walking on my lunch hour because I was too tired or busy when I got home."
—*Carolyn*

Research suggests that regular physical activity is good for you before, during, and after pregnancy. How much exercise is enough to reap the rewards? According to the Dietary Guidelines, adults require a minimum of thirty minutes of moderate-intensity exercise on most days for weight maintenance (provided that calorie intake is balanced with calories burned); sixty minutes to manage body weight and prevent gradual weight gain; and sixty to ninety minutes to maintain weight loss. There's more about exercise guidelines during pregnancy and breastfeeding in chapters 4 and 5.

It may not seem possible to squeeze one more task into your busy schedule, but living a more active lifestyle may be easier than you think. Here are some tips for making physical activity part of your everyday routine. Check with your doctor before beginning any exercise program.

- **Break it down.** Combine short bouts of activity throughout the day. For example, park your car at least a ten-minute walk away from your destination, and instantly guarantee twenty minutes of exercise; add another ten-minute walk at lunchtime, and you've got thirty minutes covered.

- **Track yourself.** Invest in a wearable device to log your steps. Work your way up to taking ten thousand steps every day, as long as your health care provider says that amount is OK for you.

- **Schedule exercise.** Treat working out like an important appointment that you must keep. If you're a "morning person," exercising early in the day is energizing, and makes it more likely that you won't miss your workout as the day goes on and you become busier.

- **Get support.** It's easier and more fun to work out with someone. Enlist a workout buddy, such as your spouse, partner, or coworker; join a walking group; or take an exercise class.

- **Have an alternative plan.** Keep exercise videos on hand or consult the Internet for a workout routine for when bad weather prevents you from walking or running outdoors or from getting to the gym. Consider investing in a treadmill or a stationary bike for inside exercise, too. Have more than one walking companion. That way, if one friend cancels, you'll still have other people to motivate you to move.

- **Mix it up.** Boredom can spell doom for your exercise routine, so find activities you enjoy. Pick at least two activities, such as walking outside, weight training, and yoga, and alternate them. Include weight training twice a week for stronger bones, toned muscles, and a more efficient metabolism.

FROM HERE TO PATERNITY: A FATHER'S PRECONCEPTION TO-DO LIST

Future dads might be under the impression that their contribution to the next generation begins and ends at conception and that mom has the remainder of the responsibility for making a healthy baby. More and more, however, research shows that both mom and dad contribute to a future child's well-being. Work together before and after the positive pregnancy test for the healthiest family possible.

Sperm is produced on a continuous basis. It takes about three months for sperm to fully develop. The number of sperm that a man has affects his ability to father a child, and so does sperm quality. There are several things fathers-to-be should do before the baby-making begins.

✓ Practice Girth Control

Large population studies show that being overweight or obese decreases sperm count. The effects seem to be inversely related—that is, the higher the body mass index, the lower the sperm count.

✓ Take a Multivitamin

Words of Motherly Wisdom

"We both needed to drop a few pounds, so my husband and I worked on weight control together before trying for a baby. Having a partner to work out with made it easier."

—*Shana*

A balanced eating plan based on whole grains, fruits, vegetables, and low-fat protein foods helps to insure that men get the nutrients necessary for making top-notch sperm. Vitamin C, zinc, and folic acid are particularly important (see chapter 3 to plan a healthy diet). Although supplements are no substitute for a healthy diet, a daily multivitamin fills in small nutrient gaps that can reduce fertility, so it is a good idea for men to take a multivitamin every day. The best multivitamin/mineral for men is one with very little or no iron that also provides 100 percent of the Daily Value for the nutrients it contains. A man's daily iron requirement is less than half that of a woman's, so men typically satisfy iron needs through food.

✓ Get a Move On

Don't wait too long to try to father a child. Age probably plays a role in fertility because sperm count declines as you get older, starting at about age thirty-five.

✓ Avoid Tobacco

If you're still smoking or chewing tobacco, do all that you can to quit as soon as possible. Tobacco use stresses sperm by leading to sperm damage, by lowering sperm count, and by diminishing sperm quality. Men who use tobacco may have a lower sperm count than those who don't smoke. Secondhand smoke also may affect male fertility.

✓ Rethink Medications and Recreational Drugs

Certain prescription and over-the-counter drugs, including those for treating hair loss, depression, and reflux disease, can impair a man's ability to father a child. Marijuana, anabolic steroids (taken to stimulate muscle strength and growth), and long-term use of opiates, including heroin and prescription medications to treat pain, can decrease the quantity and quality of sperm.

✓ Limit Alcohol Use

Drinking too much alcohol can lead to erectile dysfunction and decreased sperm production, but the link between moderate drinking and fertility in men isn't clear. If you're trying for a baby, limit alcohol to two drinks daily to be on the safer side.

✓ Stay Cool

Elevated temperatures impair sperm production and function. Sitting for long periods, wearing tight clothing, or working on a laptop computer that's perched on your lap for long stretches of time may increase the temperature in the scrotum and may slightly reduce sperm production.

WHEN YOU'RE HAVING DIFFICULTY GETTING PREGNANT: THE DIET, LIFESTYLE, AND FERTILITY CONNECTION

Perhaps you're doing everything you "should" to get pregnant, but it's not working. If you and your partner have been trying to conceive for at least a year (or six months if you're older than thirty-five), you may be experiencing infertility.

Infertility affects both women and men. According to the Centers for Disease Control and Prevention, about 12 percent of women ages fifteen to forty-four in the United States have difficulty getting pregnant or carrying a pregnancy to term. In approximately 40 percent of infertile couples, the male partner is either the sole cause or a contributing cause of infertility. There are many reasons for the infertility that affects millions of American couples, a few of which are examined in this section, but some cases of infertility cannot be explained.

Polycystic Ovary Syndrome

Ovulation disorders, including polycystic ovary syndrome, are the most common culprits in curbing female fertility. Pelvic inflammatory disease and endometriosis also cause ovulation disorders.

Polycystic ovary syndrome (PCOS) affects between one in ten and one in twenty women of childbearing age. As many as five million women in the United States may be affected. PCOS is the number-one reason for infertility in women. PCOS causes menstrual irregularities that prevent you from becoming pregnant, and it can upset hormonal balance in your body, harm your heart health, and affect your appearance. No one is exactly sure what causes PCOS, but experts suspect that family history plays a role, along with several other factors, including insulin resistance.

Many women with PCOS have difficulty using insulin, a hormone the body produces that facilitates the cells' use of glucose (energy) from the bloodstream. With too much insulin in their blood, women with PCOS produce excessive androgens, including testosterone. High levels of androgens lead to acne, excessive hair growth (including facial hair), weight gain, and problems with ovulation that impede conception.

> ### Words of Motherly Wisdom
>
> "When we went through fertility treatment, what helped me the most was when my doctor told me it wasn't our fault that we were having difficulty getting pregnant. Eventually, I gave birth to healthy twin boys."
> —Lisa H.

There is no cure for PCOS, so managing it is paramount to your health and to your chances of becoming pregnant. Treatment for PCOS should be tailored to your particular circumstances and should include a balanced, enjoyable eating plan and regular physical activity (with your doctor's approval).

Lifestyle plays a critical role in managing PCOS and promoting pregnancy. Many, but not all, women with PCOS are overweight. If you weigh too much (see page 139 for more on body weight), losing just 10 percent of your body weight—about 18 pounds for a woman who weighs 175 pounds—may help restore normal periods. Follow the MyPlate Pre-pregnancy Eating Plan in chapter 3 to help you shed some pounds. Include regular physical activity to naturally reduce blood glucose levels and make weight control easier. If you need more help, ask your doctor for a referral to a registered dietitian nutritionist (RDN) to help you develop the best eating plan for your situation.

Along with other lifestyle changes, you should not smoke cigarettes if you have PCOS. Medication may be helpful in treating PCOS. Surgery to bring on ovulation may also be the answer for some women to encourage conception.

Women with PCOS are more likely to have a mother or sister with PCOS. If you suspect that you have PCOS, see your doctor for a complete physical exam. The following are symptoms of PCOS to consider:

- Elevated insulin levels in the blood

- Infertility (inability to get pregnant) because you're not ovulating

- Cysts on the ovaries

- Acne, oily skin, or dandruff

- Infrequent menstrual periods, no menstrual periods, and/or irregular bleeding

- Hirsutism—increased hair growth on the face, chest, stomach, back, thumbs, or toes

- Weight gain or obesity, usually with extra weight around the waist

- Male-pattern baldness or thinning hair

- Skin tags—excess flaps of skin in the armpits or on the neck

- Pelvic pain

- Anxiety or depression

- Sleep apnea—when breathing stops for short periods of time while asleep

Celiac Disease

Celiac disease may be the reason why you're having trouble getting pregnant. In celiac disease, gluten—one of the proteins found in wheat, barley, and rye—triggers an overreaction by the immune system that damages the small intestine. The destruction that gluten causes reduces the body's capacity to absorb nutrients, including iron, and causes other health problems that may influence fertility and pregnancy.

One recent study estimates that 1 in 141 Americans has celiac disease, and that most cases are undiagnosed. The symptoms of celiac disease may include diarrhea, weight loss, anemia, headaches, fatigue, and an itchy, blistery skin rash. There are several hundred other signs of celiac disease, many of which are annoying and may be short-lived, such as canker sores, irregular periods, sinus pain, and sinusitis. A full and ever-expanding list can be found on the website celiac.org/symptoms.

Celiac disease may go undiagnosed for years. Some research suggests a link between untreated celiac disease and reproductive problems, such as menstrual disorders, unexplained infertility, recurrent miscarriage, and low-birth-weight babies. Celiac disease can also cause male fertility problems.

If your or your male partner's fertility problems cannot be explained, consider being screened for celiac disease. There is no cure for celiac disease, but you can manage the condition with a gluten-free eating plan and overcome any reproductive and pregnancy problems linked with celiac disease. Gluten-free diets can be low in carbohydrates, iron, zinc, folic acid, niacin, and calcium. Work closely with an RDN who specializes in celiac disease to tailor an eating plan to fit your nutritional needs before, during, and after pregnancy.

For more information about celiac disease, visit the National Institutes of Health (NIH) Celiac Disease Awareness Campaign at celiac.nih.gov.

FROM THE RECIPE FILE

See chapter 8 for delicious gluten-free recipes for smoothies, breakfast, entrees, pizza, soups, desserts, and more.

Stress

For some couples, trying to get pregnant can be stressful, especially as time passes. Women who have problems with fertility report higher levels of stress and anxiety, which in turn may contribute to infertility. Training yourself to feel calmer by using the body's own relaxation response can be helpful when tension gets the better of you. The relaxation response lowers heart rate, blood pressure, and breathing rate, allowing you to feel calmer. Feelings of calm can remain for hours.

Deep breathing and meditation are two ways to elicit the relaxation response. The book *Relaxation Revolution: The Science and Genetics of Mind Body Healing,* by Herbert Benson, MD, and William Proctor, provides instructions for eliciting the relaxation response. *Conquering Infertility: Dr. Alice Domar's Mind/Body Guide to Enhancing Fertility and Coping with Infertility,* by Alice Domar, PhD, is an excellent resource for couples having trouble getting pregnant.

A balanced diet can help to relieve stress by providing the nutrients you need to stay energized. Limit your intake of caffeine and alcohol to help ensure that you get the restful sleep you need at night, which can help you to feel calmer during the day. Regular physical activity is also a great stress reliever.

A HEALTHIER LIFE MAY IMPROVE FERTILITY

Certain lifestyle choices may improve your chances of conceiving a child. According to researchers at the Harvard T.H. Chan School of Public Health, the more healthy choices you make, the lower your chances are for ovulation disorders. An eight-year population study followed 17,544 married nurses who did not have any history of infertility. Researchers found that the women with irregular or absent ovulation—which is responsible for 18 to 30 percent of infertility—lowered their infertility risk by 80 percent by changing five or more aspects of their diet and exercise routine, as compared to women who changed none. The women with the highest fertility rates ate less trans fat and added sugar; ate more protein from vegetable sources than from animal foods; included more dietary fiber and iron; took more multivitamins; and consumed more high-fat dairy foods and fewer low-fat dairy products. Bottom line: healthy choices can't solve all cases of ovulation disorders, but they may make a difference in boosting fertility.

PREGNANCY TAKES PREPARATION

Phew! This chapter is jammed-packed with information, but you made it through! You have a better understanding of your preconception health plan, and of what you and your partner may need to do before you try to have a baby, including achieving and maintaining a healthy weight, exercising regularly, and taking a daily multivitamin.

Now, it's time to delve into carbohydrates, fat, protein, and the many other nutrients that support your health and that of your future baby. Chapter 2 is all about building your knowledge on the role of nutrition before, during, and after pregnancy.

2

Great Expectations: How Eating Healthy Food Is Good for You and Your Baby

In chapter 1, you learned about how your lifestyle and overall health can influence the chances of conceiving and of having the healthiest child possible. A balanced diet is a powerful ally before, during, and after pregnancy. Every nutrient that's good for you as an adult is good for your baby's growth, and certain nutrients are even more important during pregnancy and breastfeeding.

If you're into details, this chapter is for you. There are a lot of facts and figures ahead, but you don't need to dwell on them. Devour all the fine points now, or just skim the chapter and know that you can come back to it when you have questions. You can also skip to chapter 3, where you'll find how to put all this chapter's information together to plan healthy meals and snacks. It's up to you!

CARBOHYDRATES

Carbohydrates, a source of fuel for the body, are found in foods such as milk, yogurt, fruit, vegetables, legumes (beans), bread, cereals, pasta, rice, and other grains, as well as in cookies, cakes, and other sweets. In addition to being the body's preferred energy source, the right amount of carbohydrate in your eating plan also prevents your body from using protein for energy, which allows protein to perform its important duties, such as supporting your baby's rapid growth and development.

With the exception of fiber (more on fiber later), each form of carbohydrate provides 4 calories per gram, including the simple sugars found naturally in foods such as fruit and plain milk, added sweeteners such as table sugar, honey, and maple syrup, and the more complex carbohydrates, also known as starches, found in grain-based foods, fruits, and vegetables. The body converts the carbohydrates you eat into glucose, the fuel that it needs to keep every cell energized and functioning to its fullest potential.

Nutrition experts suggest that you consume most of your carbohydrates from foods rich in complex carbohydrates. Starch and other complex carbohydrates take longer for the body to digest, and they provide a slower and steadier energy release into the bloodstream. When you eat foods rich in simple sugars, such as table sugar and corn syrup, the carbohydrate is more readily absorbed and converted into glucose by the body, producing more immediate energy that may be followed by an energy lull. Complex carbohydrates are also preferred because they are almost always found in foods that supply vitamins, minerals, and phytonutrients (protective plant compounds) that are beneficial at all stages of life. Foods rich in complex carbohydrates include whole-grain bread, cereals, rice, pasta, vegetables, and legumes (beans). See chapter 8 for delicious and nutritious recipes for energizing quick breads, smoothies, main dishes, side dishes, desserts, and more.

Your carbohydrate needs are determined by your daily calorie requirements: 45 to 65 percent of total daily calories should come from carbohydrates. For example, you need 202 to 293 grams of carbohydrates a day on an 1,800-calorie diet; 248 to 358 grams on a 2,200-calorie diet;

and 281 to 406 grams on a 2,500-calorie diet. To get enough protein and healthy fat in your eating plan, it's best to eat about half or a bit more of your calories as carbohydrate.

When you eat the suggested number of servings of fruits, vegetables, and whole grains discussed in chapter 3, there's really no need to tally your total carbohydrate intake, but just for the record, the recommended minimum is 130 grams of carbohydrates per day when you are not pregnant, 175 grams a day when you are pregnant, and 210 grams of carbohydrate daily when breastfeeding. It's important to eat enough carbohydrate from a variety of healthy foods. Low-carbohydrate eating patterns—which typically include 60 to 130 grams of carbohydrate a day—can leave you feeling sluggish because they lack adequate energy and other nutrients.

For packaged foods, carbohydrate content is listed on the Nutrition Facts panel. But the fresh fruits and vegetables that you buy in the produce department of the grocery store don't come with food labels. Some grocery stores now post signs in the produce section listing the nutritional content of fruits and veggies. Here are some common sources of carbohydrate:

Food	Carbohydrate (grams)
Banana, large	52
Bagel, egg, 3 ounces	45
Corn, 1 cup, cooked	40
Raisins, seeded, 1/4 cup	33
Potato, medium, flesh and skin, cooked	31
Orange juice, 1 cup	28
Oatmeal, 1 cup, cooked	27
Butternut squash, 1 cup, cooked	24
Figs, dried, 1/4 cup	22
Blueberries, 1 cup, fresh	22
Black beans, 1/2 cup, cooked	20
Quinoa, 1/2 cup, cooked	20

Apple, with skin, large, raw	15
Bread, whole wheat, 1 ounce slice	14
Kiwi, 1	13
Carrots, 1 cup, cooked	13
Milk, 1% low-fat, 1 cup	12
Broccoli, 1 cup, cooked	11
Collard greens, 1 cup, cooked	11
Green beans, 1 cup, cooked	10

SUGAR

Although sugar is a simple carbohydrate, it merits its own section because it makes up a significant portion of the caloric intake of many Americans. The Dietary Guidelines recommend limiting added sugar to 10 percent or less of your daily calorie intake. That amounts to about 12 teaspoons daily, or 50 grams of added sugar, on a 2,000-calorie eating plan. The American Heart Association (AHA), which also bases their added sugar suggestions on the calorie intake necessary to achieve or maintain a healthy weight, recommends eating even less added sugar. For example, the AHA daily recommended limit is the equivalent of 8 teaspoons (32 grams) of added sugar on a 2,000-calorie eating plan; 12 teaspoons (48 grams) on a 2,400-calorie plan; or 14 teaspoons (56 grams) on a 2,600-calorie plan.

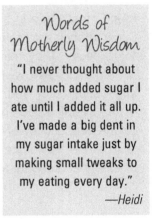

Words of Motherly Wisdom

"I never thought about how much added sugar I ate until I added it all up. I've made a big dent in my sugar intake just by making small tweaks to my eating every day."
—*Heidi*

No matter which expert guidelines you choose to follow, it's important to remember that most foods with added sugar, such as soda, candy, and cookies, offer little, if any, nutrition. What's more, added sugar contributes calories. For example, equal portions of certain sugary breakfast cereals can have many more calories than their no-sugar-added counterparts. In addition, excess sugar may increase the risk for obesity, heart disease, and type 2 diabetes.

ALTERNATIVE SWEETENERS AND PREGNANCY: A GOOD MATCH?

There's a lot to consider when choosing a sweetener during pregnancy. Generally speaking, it's safe to use most sweeteners, such as sucralose and aspartame, when pregnant and breastfeeding, but saccharin is not considered safe during pregnancy because it is capable of crossing the placenta and lingering in your baby's tissues. Limited research shows that popular sugar alternatives show up in breast milk, but the effects on baby are not well understood. The Food and Drug Administration has approved rebaudioside A (Reb A), one of the many compounds in stevia leaves, as a sweetener, but has not approved other forms of stevia, such as whole-leaf stevia and crude extracts. Look for Reb A on stevia packages to be sure of what form of stevia is contained in the package. Sugar alcohols, such as sorbitol and xylitol, are another category of sweeteners used in place of added sugars. Sugar alcohols are found most often in sugar-free candies, cookies, and chewing gums. Sugar alcohols are slightly lower in calories than sugar and don't promote tooth decay. They may cause gas and bloating, however. Pregnancy is a time to make wise food choices, so if you're going overboard on sugar substitutes you may need to take a closer look at what you're eating overall. Foods made with sugar substitutes are not necessarily calorie-free, and lower-calorie foods sweetened with sugar substitutes, such as diet carbonated soft drinks, may not provide appreciable levels of essential nutrients for pregnancy.

While you may need to cut back on added sugar, there is no need to go completely sugar-free. The recommendations from the Dietary Guidelines and the AHA target *added* sugar, not the natural sugars found in foods such as fruit, fruit juice, vegetables, and plain dairy foods (called lactose). Added sugar can be part of a balanced eating pattern, and small amounts of sugar added to healthy foods such as plain yogurt and plain oatmeal make it more likely you'll eat them. Limiting or reducing foods with lots of added sugar, particularly sugary drinks, makes room in your diet for more nutrient-rich food choices. For example, sipping low-fat milk instead of soda helps to satisfy protein, calcium, and vitamin D requirements. Choosing fruit instead of cookies supplies more fiber, vitamins, minerals, and phytonutrients (see more about phytonutrients on page 87).

REALITY CHECK: THE JUICY DETAILS

You won't find added sugar in 100 percent fruit juice because it derives its sweet taste from naturally occurring sugars. Juice contains vitamins, minerals, and phytonutrients (beneficial plant compounds), but it lacks the fiber found in whole fruit. Juice is useful for helping to satisfying your daily fruit and fluid requirements. Just remember that it contains calories, so drink it in moderation.

Being aware of your daily sugar allowance in teaspoons and in grams is helpful for curbing added sugar intake. Total carbohydrate content is expressed in grams on the Nutrition Facts panel, and added sugars will be included on most Nutrition Facts panels by July of 2018. To help you make more informed food choices, the amount of added sugar will be listed in grams and as a percentage of the Daily Value for a 2,000-calorie eating plan.

Added sugar goes by different names. The following is a list of the many names of sugar that you may find in an ingredient list. Use it to help limit your intake of foods with added sugar:

- agave syrup
- anhydrous dextrose
- brown sugar
- cane juice
- confectioner's powdered sugar
- corn syrup
- corn syrup solids
- crystal dextrose
- dextrose
- evaporated cane juice
- evaporated corn sweetener
- fruit juice concentrate
- fruit nectar
- fructose

- glucose
- high-fructose corn syrup (HFCS)
- honey
- invert sugar
- lactose
- liquid fructose
- malt syrup
- maltose
- maple syrup

- molasses
- nectars (e.g., peach nectar, pear nectar)
- pancake syrup
- raw sugar
- sorghum syrup
- sucrose
- sugar
- sugar cane juice
- white granulated sugar

When you're craving sugar, managing your desire for something sweet can be challenging. Here's how to satisfy your sweet tooth and include important nutrients:

- **Avoid sugary beverages.** Nearly half of all the added sugar we consume comes from sugary soda, sports drinks, energy drinks, and other sweet beverages. Drink plain or carbonated unsweetened flavored water, or fat-free or low-fat milk instead. Skip sweet coffee drinks and opt for unsweetened versions with your own added milk and a small amount of sugar or honey. Fill a tall glass with cold seltzer water, and add just a splash of 100 percent fruit juice. Reduce the sugar content of hot cocoa and chocolate milk by making your own instead of buying it premade.

- **Minimize sweet treats.** Cookies, candy, snack bars, and other sweets can supply a significant amount of added sugar in your diet. Put these foods in the "occasional" category, and reach for treats in smaller portions, such as a mini cupcake or a fun-size candy bar, and take the time to savor them. For most people, the first few bites are the most pleasurable, but if you're not satisfied with just a small portion, you may want to avoid sweet treats entirely to keep yourself from overeating them.

- **Buy plain yogurt (regular or Greek) and mix in your own flavors.** Stir a teaspoon of low-sugar fruit preserves, honey, or molasses into 8 ounces of plain yogurt. You may also enjoy plain yogurt with fresh or frozen fruit.

- **Rely on fruit for sweetness.** Swap syrup on pancakes and waffles for applesauce or other pureed fruit. Whip up a smoothie with ripe fruit, ice, and milk or plain Greek yogurt.

- **Skip the sugared cereals.** Purchase no-sugar cereals, such as plain oatmeal, and add fresh or dried fruit for sweetness. If you don't want to give up sugared cereals entirely, mix higher-sugar cereals with lower-sugar (less than 5 grams of sugar per serving), higher-fiber varieties to cut sugar consumption.

- **Modify recipes.** When making muffins and other quick breads, cut the amount of sugar called for in the recipe by at least one-third.

- **Do not keep sweet treats in the house.** Why tempt yourself? It's easier to manage sugar intake when candy, cake, and cookies are not calling your name from the kitchen.

- **Limit prepared foods and condiments that may contain added sugars.** These can include barbecue sauce, ketchup, pasta sauce, and breads. Compare brands by reading the Nutrient Facts panels and lists of ingredients, and search for those with the lowest sugar content.

FROM THE RECIPE FILE

You won't believe that this Fruit and Nut Bread has no added sugar!
Fruit provides all the sweetness you need. See page 236 for the recipe.

DIETARY FIBER

Fiber contributes few if any calories (energy) to your diet because your body doesn't digest and absorb it. That doesn't diminish its contributions to good health, however.

Fiber helps to keep you fuller longer, which is beneficial when you're trying to control your weight. It also plays a role in lowering blood cholesterol levels and keeping blood glucose concentrations in a normal range.

Fiber is helpful for preventing and relieving constipation, which is a common side effect of pregnancy. Large doses of supplemental iron may also cause constipation. Fiber adds bulk to soften stools, making them easier to pass. Avoiding constipation helps you prevent hemorrhoids, which can result during pregnancy from straining to move your bowels.

Fiber requirements relate to calorie needs, and they change just slightly with impending motherhood. Generally speaking, nonpregnant women need 25 grams of fiber daily, pregnant women need 28 grams, and nursing women need 29 grams. Fiber absorbs many times its weight in fluid, so it's important to consume a sufficient amount of water (from fluids, fruits, and vegetables) each day to keep your digestive tract in working order (see "Fluids," on page 52, for the proper amounts).

Look under "Dietary Fiber" on the Nutrition Facts panel of food labels for the fiber content of packaged foods. Many foods with fiber, such as fruit and vegetables, lack labels, so refer to the list below for their fiber levels.

Food	Fiber (grams)
Navy beans, 1/2 cup, cooked	10
Lentils, 1/2 cup, cooked	8
Black beans, 1/2 cup, cooked	8
Garbanzo beans, 1/2 cup, cooked	8
White beans, 1/2 cup, cooked	6
Pear, 1 medium	6
Avocado, 1/2 cup	5
Soybeans, 1/2 cup, cooked	5
Peas, 1/2 cup, cooked	4
Chia seeds, 1 tablespoon	4
Apple, medium, with skin	4

Raspberries, $^1/_2$ cup	4
Potato, medium, with skin, baked	4
Sweet potato, medium, flesh only, baked	4
Almonds, 1 ounce	4
Broccoli, $^1/_2$ cup, cooked	3
Orange, 1 medium	3
Banana, 1 medium	3
Quinoa, $^1/_2$ cup, cooked	3

FROM THE RECIPE FILE

Peanut, Raspberry, Banana, and Oats Smoothie Bowl is a delicious way to include about half of your daily fiber needs along with 29 grams of protein. See page 230 for the recipe.

PROTEIN

Protein is the structural component of every part of your body and your baby's body. Pregnant women need dietary protein to support the production of new cells, enzymes, and the hormones that promote and regulate life. Adequate protein during pregnancy helps your baby to grow fully; to develop hair, fingernails, skin, and organs; and to achieve a healthy birth weight. Protein also plays a role in keeping fluid balance in check. Fluid balance is important to help prevent pregnancy swelling and for maintaining normal blood pressure.

The proteins that are found in your body, such as in cells, hormones, and muscle, are constructed from a series of building blocks called *amino acids*. Although protein supplies 4 calories per gram, the body needs protein from foods primarily for the amino acids they contain, rather than for using protein as energy. The nitrogen that food protein provides is important, too, because nitrogen is necessary for cell growth and repair.

Both quantity and quality count in meeting your protein needs. Animal and plant foods provide amino acids, but the protein in animal foods—such as beef, poultry, pork, eggs, milk, and seafood—is different from nearly all plant protein. Animal foods are rich in all the amino acids that the body is unable to make on its own, known as indispensable amino acids (IAAs) or essential amino acids (EAAs). Soy foods and quinoa are the only two plant foods that contain all the IAAs. You must get the IAAs you need from food.

Even though they are nutritious, plant foods, such as nearly all legumes and grains, lack adequate amounts of one or more of the IAAs. Women who avoid or eat few animal foods should aim to include a variety of protein-rich plant products such as tofu, tempeh, soy beverages, edamame (fresh soybeans), quinoa, legumes, and nuts as part of a balanced diet in order to get the right mix of amino acids every day, particularly during pregnancy and breastfeeding. If you avoid all animal foods, it would be a good idea to consult a registered dietitian nutritionist (RDN) to plan a diet that meets your needs for protein and other nutrients before, during, and after pregnancy.

Protein needs are related to your body weight, and they can vary based on physical activity. The recommendation is .36 grams of protein per pound of body weight per day. For example, a 135-pound woman who isn't expecting a child should consume at least 49 grams of protein daily, and more if she is physically active. Women in the first trimester require the same amount of protein as nonpregnant women because the baby doesn't increase in size much in early pregnancy. Once the second trimester starts, protein requirements rise by 25 grams a day and stay that high throughout pregnancy and breastfeeding. That means our 135-pound woman would need a minimum of 74 grams of protein every day—about the amount found in a combination of 3 ounces of cooked chicken, one egg, 1 cup of yogurt, 16 ounces of milk, and 2 tablespoons of peanut butter. If you are pregnant with twins, your daily protein needs increase by 50 grams. It is a good idea to bump up your protein intake as soon as you find out you're expecting more than one child, and not wait until the second trimester.

Protein does not come in prenatal vitamin pills or regular multivitamin supplements, so plan on filling your daily quota with food. Refer to the following list to keep your protein intake up to par.

Food	Protein (grams)
Chicken breast, boneless, skinless, 3 ounces, cooked	27
Tuna, light, canned, drained, 3 ounces	25
Pork tenderloin, 3 ounces, roasted	22
Salmon, Atlantic, 3 ounces, cooked	22
Beef, 95% lean, 3 ounces, cooked	21
Soybeans (edamame), 1/2 cup, dry roasted	20
Yogurt, Greek, plain, fat-free, 5.6 ounces	17
Cottage cheese, low-fat, 1/2 cup	14
Yogurt, plain, low-fat, 8 ounces	12
Yogurt, fruit-flavored, low-fat, 1 cup	11
Tofu, 1/2 cup, raw	10
Lentils, 1/2 cup, cooked	9
Peanut butter, 2 tablespoons	9
Milk, 1% low-fat, 1 cup	9
Milk, whole, 1 cup	8
Soy beverage, 1 cup	8
Black beans, canned, drained, 1/2 cup	7
Almond butter, 2 tablespoons	7
Cheddar cheese, 1 ounce	6
Egg, 1 large	6
Pistachios, 1 ounce	6
Garbanzo beans, canned, drained, 1/2 cup	6
Quinoa, 1/2 cup, cooked	4

FAT

Fat is a three-letter word, but it might as well be a four-letter curse for all the respect it gets. Fat serves up more than twice the calories (9 per gram) of carbohydrates or protein, which is why many people try to limit it in the name of weight control. You may be surprised to learn that health experts say fat is an essential nutrient to include in a balanced eating plan, whether you are pregnant, planning on becoming pregnant, or breastfeeding a baby. Quality counts, however.

The body requires dietary fat for several reasons. First, fat provides energy. In fact, it would be very difficult to satisfy your calorie needs without fat, especially during pregnancy and breastfeeding, and it would be hard to stay healthy. That's because some types of fat supply essential fatty acids (EFAs), compounds that support your health and are absolutely necessary for your child's development. The body cannot produce the EFAs—linoleic acid and alpha-linolenic acid—so it must get them from food. (Infants get EFAs from breast milk and from infant formula.) Second, fat promotes the body's ability to absorb vitamins A, D, E, and K—known as the fat-soluble vitamins—and helps to get them where they need to go in the body. In addition, fat provides flavor and eating satisfaction.

Fat Facts: Saturated, Unsaturated, and Trans Fat

The fat in foods is categorized as *saturated* and *unsaturated*. These two types of fat occur naturally in foods. The majority of another type of fat we eat, called *trans fat,* is manufactured, but some trans fat is naturally occurring. Foods often contain a mixture of fat types, which are listed on the Nutrition Facts panel of packaged food products. (As is the case with produce, most of the meat you'll find in the refrigerated meat case at your grocery store isn't required to have a Nutrition Facts panel. The exception is packaged processed meat such as cold cuts and bacon.)

Animal foods—such as fatty meats and full-fat dairy foods like cheese, ice cream, and whole milk—supply most of the saturated fat in the typical American diet. Coconut oil, palm oil, palm kernel oil, and cocoa butter, which are all used widely in packaged foods such as cookies, crackers, and candy, are highly saturated fats, too.

Saturated fat is scorned for its role in promoting heart disease. For many people, eating excess saturated fat contributes to elevated cholesterol levels and clogged arteries. Clogged arteries block blood flow and increase the risk of heart attack and stroke. Pregnant or not, you don't need any saturated fat in your diet because your body produces all that it requires.

To help protect your heart, the Dietary Guidelines suggest limiting your daily intake of saturated fat to 10 percent of calories or less, which is about 22 grams on a 2,000-calorie eating plan. Saturated fat content is clearly listed on most food labels, and that's helpful for determining food choices.

REALITY CHECK: YOU DON'T HAVE TO SACK SATURATED FAT

There's no need to completely avoid foods with saturated fat. Foods such as meat and cheese contain protein, vitamins, and minerals that are vital to a growing baby and a healthy mother, and they taste good, too! Consider consuming smaller portions of foods higher in saturated fats or eating them less often to keep your saturated fat intake within the recommended range.

Trace amounts of naturally occurring trans fat can be found in meats and full-fat dairy foods, but, by far, the majority of the trans fat in our food supply is the result of hydrogenation, a process that creates a firmer, tastier product from unsaturated fats. Hydrogenation increases the stability of unsaturated fat, making it ideal to use in processed foods, which require fats with a long shelf life to prevent spoilage.

Like saturated fat, trans fat contributes to clogged arteries and more. There is no dietary requirement for trans fat, but it's nearly impossible to avoid it completely. Most packaged food is required to list trans fat content on the food label, but there is a hitch. A serving of food can contain some trans fat even when the amount of trans fat listed is zero ("trans-free"). That's because it's permissible by law to list the trans fat content of a serving of food as zero if it contains up to half a gram.

Although many manufacturers have reduced or eliminated the trans fat in their products in recent years, this man-made fat may still be found in small amounts in some stick margarine, shortening, frozen pizzas, canned frosting, french fries and other fast foods, cookies, crackers, granola bars, and microwave popcorn. Occasional intake of foods with minimal trans fat is not considered problematic, but experts want you to eat very little trans fat, if any, for the sake of your heart. The most effective way to avoid trans fat is to check the ingredient list on food labels for "partially hydrogenated oil," which alerts you that the product contains trans fat, even if the Nutrition Facts panel says it has none. Consuming foods with partially hydrogenated oils on a regular basis can add up to excess trans fat intake. Limit trans fat with a balanced eating plan that includes minimally processed foods, including fast foods and bakery items. Rely on canola, olive, and sunflower oils for cooking, baking, and flavoring foods.

Trans fat is a nutritional bad guy, but there is good news about it. Avoiding trans fat will get easier. In 2015, the FDA ruled that partially hydrogenated oils (PHO) will not be allowed in processed foods after June 18, 2018, unless they are otherwise approved by FDA.

Unsaturated fats are more desirable because they are considered heart-healthy. Monounsaturated fat is the primary fat in olive oil, canola oil, sesame oil, avocados, nuts, peanuts, and peanut butter. Polyunsaturated fat is found in the greatest amounts in corn oil, cottonseed oil, safflower oil, sunflower seeds, flaxseed, and seafood. Oils are favored as part of a healthy eating plan because they are a major source of EFAs and vitamin E. Omega-3 fats are a type of polyunsaturated fat found in higher levels in fattier fish—for example, salmon, trout, herring, tuna, shrimp, and mackerel—and in certain other foods, including walnuts and flaxseeds.

Fish and Omega-3 Fats

Fish and shellfish, as mentioned above, supply omega-3 fats. These unsaturated fats are good for your heart, and for your baby, too. Seafood is the best natural source of a certain type of omega-3 fat called docosahexaenoic acid (DHA) that plays a central role in your child's brain development during pregnancy, infancy, and the first few years of life. Seafood is also a source of eicosapentaenoic acid (EPA), which isn't directly involved in brain development but which may help DHA cross the placenta. It benefits mom's health, too.

DHA is the dominant fat in the brain. It's part of every brain cell your child has or will have. Research shows that DHA helps to develop your baby's brain, particularly from about the twenty-fourth week of pregnancy on, when his or her brain is developing rapidly. DHA also accumulates in the retina, located at the back of each eye, where it contributes to vision. The retina has been called the "window to the world" because it's involved in registering what you see and transmitting those images to the brain for processing.

Your body can store DHA, so it's important to get enough at all stages of life. The DHA you have in reserve and the DHA you consume from foods during pregnancy and breastfeeding helps your baby get the DHA he or she requires. (If you don't breastfeed, your baby can get DHA in most brands of infant formula, although the levels vary.) Adults and children of all ages can convert alpha-linolenic acid—the essential fat found in walnuts, flax, and other foods—to DHA, but only an estimated 10 percent is actually formed into DHA.

A recent review of dozens of studies concluded that pregnant and breastfeeding women should consume at least 200 milligrams (mg) of DHA daily, which is in keeping with recommendations from health organizations around the world. Generally speaking, many women do not consume enough DHA during the childbearing years. DHA is found almost exclusively in seafood, and some fish, including the fattier varieties such as salmon and canned white tuna, have more DHA than others. Seafood also supplies protein, vitamins, and minerals that you and your baby need.

Eating the suggested amount of lower-mercury fish, such as canned tuna, salmon, and shrimp, makes it easier to meet your DHA needs. The DGA recommends that all adults consume at least two fish meals (8 ounces total) of a variety of fish every week, and that pregnant and breastfeeding women include even more; they should eat two to three low-mercury fish meals (8 to 12 ounces total) weekly as part of a balanced eating plan. On average, pregnant women eat less than half a serving (2 ounces of seafood) per week, or just 25 percent of the suggested minimum intake. See chapter 6 for more about the best choices for lower mercury fish.

FROM THE RECIPE FILE

Tuna Burgers with Smashed Avocado and Tomato (page 275)
is an easy-to-prepare fish dish loaded with beneficial omega-3 fats
as well as several other nutrients, including vitamin D,
the importance of which is explained in detail on page 59.

Preformed DHA is found naturally in seafood. It can also be obtained from dietary supplements and fortified foods, which are great ways to include the DHA you need every day if you don't eat fish or don't eat the recommended two to three seafood meals weekly. Rely on seafood, fortified foods, and supplements to meet your DHA needs.

Food	DHA (mg)
Salmon, Atlantic, farmed, 3 ounces, cooked	1,238
Salmon, Atlantic, wild, 3 ounces, cooked	1,215
Tuna, white, canned, drained, 3 ounces	535
Prenatal multivitamins with DHA	200
Tuna, light, canned, drained, 3 ounces	167
Tilapia, 3 ounces, cooked	113
Eggland's Best Eggs, 1 large	57
Silk DHA Omega-3 Soy Milk, 1 cup	32
Horizon Organic DHA Omega-3 Milk, 1 cup	32

FLUIDS

You know that water is essential, but did you know that it's a nutrient? Water is just as important as carbohydrates, protein, fat, and the dozens of other nutrients your body needs. You might say that water is the most essential part of your diet, given that without water you'd survive just a few days.

Water keeps your body temperature in the normal range for good health. It's part of the transportation system that carries nutrients and waste around, and out of, the body. Water moistens bodily tissues, keeping them in good working condition, and it cushions and protects your developing baby. Water also serves as the basis of breast milk.

Before you conceive, you should get about nine 8-ounce cups of fluid, including plain water, a day. Pregnant women need about thirteen 8-ounce cups of fluid daily, and nursing women need about sixteen 8-ounce cups. (One cup of liquid equals 8 "fluid" ounces.) You will require more water at every stage of life if you are physically active.

Plain water is preferable, but if it's not your beverage of choice, then coffee, tea, milk, juice, and other soft drinks, such as regular or diet carbonated beverages, can fill the void because they count toward your fluid quota. However, don't overdo it on calorie-containing beverages, such as carbonated soft drinks and 100 percent fruit juices. Too many sugary soft drinks can cause weight gain and take the place of other, more nutritious beverages. Whole fruits and vegetables are brimming with water, and they also provide fiber, vitamins, and minerals.

CAFFEINE

Caffeine is a stimulant that slightly increases blood pressure and heart rate and makes you feel more alert. Perhaps that's why caffeine is so popular! Too much caffeine may cause you to feel jittery and have problems concentrating, but just the right amount can perk you up and help you be more productive.

Once you're pregnant, you may need to reconsider your caffeine consumption. According to the March of Dimes, it takes your body longer to process caffeine after you've conceived. Caffeine can cross the placenta, but it's unclear whether that harms a developing child. There have been reports that excess caffeine can cause miscarriage and restrict a baby's growth during pregnancy, but the research is not conclusive. Most experts agree that moderate amounts of caffeine seem to be safe during pregnancy. Until we have more research about the effects of caffeine on a baby's growth and development, it's best to limit your intake to

200 milligrams daily, say the March of Dimes, the American College of Obstetricians and Gynecologists, and other expert health organizations.

REALITY CHECK:
TIRED MOM CRAVES CAFFEINE

You're exhausted and you could really use a cup of coffee to keep you going. According to the American Academy of Pediatrics, it's safe for women to consume small amounts of caffeine while breastfeeding. Remember, however, that caffeine gets into breast milk. Caffeine from any source could make for an irritable infant or one who has trouble sleeping, and, as a tired new mom, you don't want that!

Coffee is the main source of caffeine in the United States. Plain coffee offers several health perks that may surprise you. We Americans drink so much coffee that it's our diet's leading source of antioxidants, a class of compounds that help protect cells against everyday damage. Coffee also contains small amounts of the minerals potassium and magnesium, as well as niacin (one of the B vitamins) and vitamin E. If you take your coffee with milk, you get additional protein, calcium, and vitamin D; a latte made with fat-free milk has as much of these nutrients as a glass of milk. If you avoid cow's milk, have the latte with fortified soy milk for extra nutrition. Although plain coffee and coffee drinks made with fat-free and low-fat milk can be beneficial in reasonable amounts, take care with coffee shop add-ins, such as syrups and whipped cream, which can contribute high levels of added sugar and hundreds of calories to your drink. Add flavor with a sprinkle of ground cinnamon or cocoa powder instead of sugar and whipped cream.

Words of Motherly Wisdom

"Giving up caffeine completely wasn't working for me when I was pregnant with my third [child]. I had one cup of coffee a day, and it really helped me deal with my other two children!"

—Meghan

Caffeine Content

Coffee may be the primary caffeine source in the United States, but caffeine shows up in many other common beverages and foods, too. Many caffeine-containing foods and beverages declare their caffeine content on the label. Some pain-relief and cold medicines contain caffeine, and the amount is listed on the label. If you're pregnant, talk to your health care provider before taking any medicine, particularly one containing caffeine. Herbal products, which are generally not recommended during pregnancy, may also contain caffeine. See page 24 for more on caffeine intake before pregnancy.

Rely on the following list to calculate the amount of caffeine in your beverages and food, and keep your daily intake under the recommended 200 mg during pregnancy.

Product	Caffeine (mg)
Coffee	
Starbucks Brewed Coffee, grande, 16 ounces	330
Starbucks Double Shot on Ice, grande, 16 ounces	225
Starbucks Iced Brewed Coffee, grande, 16 ounces	190
Starbucks Caffe Mocha, grande, 16 ounces	175
Coffee, brewed, generic, 16 ounces, on average	170
Starbucks Iced Coffee, grande, 16 ounces	65
Coffee, brewed, generic, decaffeinated, 12 ounces, on average	2–10
Tea	
Starbucks Tazo Green Tea Latte, grande, 16 ounces	80
Snapple, Lemon (regular and diet versions), 16 ounces	62
Tea, black, brewed, 8 ounces	55
Starbucks Tazo Chai Tea Latte, grande, 16 ounces	50
Arizona Iced Tea, black, 20 ounces	30
Arizona Iced Tea, green, 16 ounces	15

Soft Drinks

Mountain Dew, regular or diet, 12 ounces	54
Starbucks Refreshers, 12 ounces	50
Diet Coke, 12 ounces	47
Dr. Pepper, regular or diet, 12 ounces	42
Pepsi, 12 ounces	38
Diet Pepsi, 12 ounces	36
Coca-Cola Classic, 12 ounces	35
Barq's Root Beer, 12 ounces	23
7-Up, regular or diet, 12 ounces	0
Fanta, all flavors, 12 ounces	0
Fresca, all flavors, 12 ounces	0
Mug Root Beer, regular or diet, 12 ounces	0
Sierra Mist, regular or sugar-free, 12 ounces	0
Sprite, regular or diet, 12 ounces	0
Barq's Diet Root Beer, 12 ounces	0

Energy Drinks

Bang Energy Drink, 16 ounces	357
Spike Shooter, 8.4 ounces	300
Amp Energy Cherry Blast, 16 ounces	160
Monster Energy, 16 ounces	160
Red Bull, 8.3 ounces	76
Red Bull, sugar-free, 8.3 ounces	75
Aquafina Alive Energize, 8 ounces	46

Miscellaneous

Stay Alert gum, 1 piece	100
Coffee-flavored ice cream, 8 ounces	58
Hershey's Special Dark Chocolate Bar, 1.5 ounces	20
Hershey's Chocolate Bar, 1.55 ounces	9

Hershey's Kisses, 9 pieces	9
Hot cocoa or chocolate milk, homemade, 8 ounces	5

Sources: Company information; JAMA Patient Page. Energy Drinks.
http://jama.jamanetwork.com/article.aspx?articleid=1487122.

FROM THE RECIPE FILE

Mocha Java Smoothie (page 224) powers you up
with protein and carbohydrate, not caffeine.

VITAMINS

Carbohydrates, protein, and fat supply fuel for cells, but these nutrients
would be out of a job if it weren't for the vitamins that help your body
use the energy they provide.

Vitamin A

Vitamin A is best known for its role in promoting optimal vision, but it
does much more than that. Vitamin A makes possible the growth and
good health of cells and tissues all over the body.

Vitamin A is actually a group of compounds that are important to
reproduction, vision, and immunity. During pregnancy, your child needs
vitamin A for cell division and for cell differentiation, which occurs
during the first trimester, when the body decides which cells will become
part of your baby's brain, muscle, bones, blood, and all other tissues.

Vitamin A comes in two forms. Retinol, or the vitamin A that's ready
to use by the body, is found most often in animal foods, such as liver
and fortified milk, and in dietary supplements. Beta-carotene, alpha-car-
otene, and beta-cryptoxanthin are carotenoids (plant compounds) that
the body is capable of converting to vitamin A. Brightly colored fruits
and vegetables, including cantaloupe, sweet potatoes, and broccoli, offer
carotenoids. Dietary supplements, including multivitamins and prenatal
multivitamins, also contain carotenoids.

Although many Americans could use more carotenoids in their diet, studies suggest that few people are deficient in total vitamin A. However, you can have too much of a good thing. Excessive amounts of retinol, typically from dietary supplements or acne medications, during early pregnancy can lead to birth defects. See chapter 1 for more on vitamin A.

Daily Needs

The requirements for vitamin A are listed in micrograms (mcg) of retinol activity equivalents (RAE) to account for the different biological activities of retinol and for the carotenoids that become vitamin A in the body. Food and dietary supplement labels list vitamin A in international units (IU). To do the conversion: 1 RAE equals 3.3 IU, although it's not necessary to calculate the vitamin A you get from foods. Here's what you need every day:

Nonpregnant woman, 14 to 50 years old: 700 mcg RAE (2,310 IU)

Pregnant, 14 to 18 years old: 750 mcg RAE (2,475 IU)

Pregnant, 19 to 50 years old: 770 mcg RAE (2,541 IU)

Breastfeeding, 14 to 18 years old: 1,200 mcg RAE (3,960 IU)

Breastfeeding, 19 to 50 years old: 1,300 mcg RAE (4,290 IU)

Very high levels of preformed vitamin A are linked to birth defects and other health problems. Do not consume more than 2,800 mcg of preformed vitamin A (9,333 IU) if you're between fourteen and eighteen years old and pregnant, and no more than 3,000 mcg (10,000 IU) of preformed vitamin A at any other time during your childbearing years.

Top Food Sources

Food	Vitamin A (mcg RAE)
Sweet potato, 1/2 cup flesh, baked	701
Spinach, 1/2 cup, cooked	573
Carrots, 1/2 cup, chopped, raw	459

Milk, fat-free, 8 ounces	149
Cantaloupe, $1/2$ cup, cubed	135
Fortified breakfast cereals, 1 serving	127–149
Egg, 1 large	75

Vitamin D

Calcium might generate the most buzz for building strong bones, but it is nearly useless without vitamin D. Vitamin D is necessary for absorbing calcium from food and dietary supplements. Vitamin D also directs the movement of calcium into and out of bones, bolstering skeletal strength and allowing a healthy concentration of calcium in your bloodstream, which promotes a regular heartbeat and normal muscle movement.

Vitamin D is a rarity among nutrients because your body makes it on its own. Exposure to strong sunshine triggers vitamin D production in the skin. The liver, kidneys, and cells in several other parts of the body convert vitamin D to its active form. Extra vitamin D is stored in your liver and body fat for future use.

In theory, your body can make all the vitamin D you need for the entire year during the months when the sun's rays are the strongest. In reality, many women do not produce enough vitamin D. Limited sun exposure can influence the levels of this vitamin in your body, even if you live in a southern climate where the sun is stronger for more months during the year. Multiple factors—including staying indoors and using sunscreen that has a sun protection factor (SPF) of 8 or above—block the sun's ultraviolet B rays that generate vitamin D in the skin. Women with darker skin, especially those who live in northern climates, where the sun is too weak to make vitamin D for half of the year or more, may be at particular risk for low vitamin D levels. Darker skin contains more melanin. Melanin provides color to skin, but it also blocks vitamin D production. There are so

Words of Motherly Wisdom

"To get the vitamin D and calcium I needed, I made chocolate milk in a water bottle. Shaking the milk instead of stirring made it taste like a milkshake!"

—Robin

many ways to affect sun exposure that it's not possible for experts to come up with general guidelines for getting adequate strong sunshine to make enough vitamin D for the entire year. In addition, few foods naturally provide vitamin D. To get the vitamin D you need, it's a good idea year-round to consume foods with natural and added vitamin D and dietary supplements that contain a form of vitamin D called vitamin D3.

Get into the habit of maintaining beneficial levels of vitamin D in your body to help yourself and your future child. Studies done with female animals suggest that vitamin D plays a role in fertility. A study published in the *Journal of Clinical Endocrinology and Metabolism* found that women who are deficient in vitamin D are half as likely to conceive using in vitro fertilization compared with women without vitamin D deficiency.

Daily Needs

Whether or not you're pregnant or breastfeeding, you need at least 600 IU of vitamin D every day from age fourteen to age seventy. Some research suggests that overweight people are at risk for vitamin D deficiency and may need more vitamin D in their diets. Certain vitamin D experts recommend higher amounts than the Recommended Dietary Allowances (listed below). Limit vitamin D intake to the suggested upper limit of 4,000 IU per day.

SHOULD YOU BE TESTED FOR VITAMIN D?

Many women don't get enough vitamin D before, during, and after pregnancy. You can't tell that your vitamin D levels are low without a blood test. While there isn't enough scientific evidence to recommend for or against testing every woman's vitamin D level before she conceives, it makes sense to be tested if you're at risk for low vitamin D. If you're pregnant and have a low blood vitamin D level, you may need to take 1,000 to 2,000 IU daily to bring it up to normal.

Top Food Sources

With the exception of certain fish and eggs, few foods naturally supply vitamin D. Fortified foods, including milk, soy beverages, yogurt, and 100 percent orange juice, help to satisfy your need for this vital vitamin.

Food	Vitamin D (IU)
Salmon, sockeye, 3 ounces, cooked	570
Salmon, pink, canned, 3 ounces	492
Tuna, light, canned, drained, 3 ounces	216
Soy milk, fortified, all flavors, unsweetened, 8 ounces	119
Orange juice, fortified, 8 ounces	100
Milk, fortified, 1% low-fat, 8 ounces	98
Yogurt, fortified, 5 ounces	74
Egg, 1 large	41
Cereal, ready-to-eat, fortified, 3/4 to 1 cup	varies

Vitamin E

The body's cells are under constant attack from free radicals, which are unstable forms of oxygen that roam the body looking to make trouble. Free radicals are the results of normal, everyday metabolism, but they can be deadly to cells by destroying cell membranes.

Oxidative stress is the term that experts use to describe the chaos created by free radicals. You can't escape free radicals, but you can limit their production by avoiding (as much as possible) smog and other air pollutants, cigarette smoking, secondhand smoke, and prolonged exposure to sunlight (ultraviolet rays).

As part of a healthy diet, vitamin E is one of the body's best weapons against daily oxidative stress. By donating part of itself to a free radical, vitamin E turns an unruly, hostile compound into a harmless substance, and the free radical becomes incapable of destruction.

Vitamin E is garnering attention for another kind of defense: its ability to fend off oxidative damage to LDL cholesterol, the "bad" cholesterol. It might seem strange to want to protect a compound known to clog arteries, but when LDL cholesterol is oxidized by free radicals, it becomes stickier and more likely to form blockages, boosting the risk of heart disease and stroke. Vitamin E can also prevent blood cells from sticking to one another and to the blood vessels in which they travel, helping to promote clear and flexible blood vessels that allow the passage of oxygen-rich blood to your heart and, when you're pregnant, to the placenta, too.

Vitamin E is a fat-soluble vitamin, so it's mostly found in higher-fat foods, such as vegetable oils, vegetable oil spreads, nuts, and seeds. There are eight forms of vitamin E in foods, but one, alpha-tocopherol, is considered superior. Though important to your health, the other seven forms of vitamin E cannot meet the body's vitamin E needs. In fact, alpha-tocopherol is so potent that the recommended dietary allowance for vitamin E is based on the body's requirement for alpha-tocopherol.

Daily Needs

Nonpregnant woman: 15 mg of alpha-tocopherol

Pregnant, all ages: 15 mg of alpha-tocopherol

Breastfeeding, all ages: 19 mg of alpha-tocopherol

Pregnant or breastfeeding: Limit intake of alpha-tocopherol to 800 mg if 14 to 18 years old and to 1,000 mg if 19 to 50 years old

Top Food Sources

Food	Vitamin E (as alpha-tocopherol, in mg)
Almond butter, 2 tablespoons	8
Almonds, 1 ounce (24 kernels), raw or roasted	7
Sunflower seeds, 1 ounce, roasted	7
Peanut butter, smooth, 2 tablespoons	6
Sunflower oil, 1 tablespoon	6
Safflower oil, 1 tablespoon	5
Wheat germ, 1/4 cup	5
Hazelnuts, 1 ounce, roasted	4

Spinach, 1 cup, cooked	4
Avocado, 1	3
Peanuts, 1 ounce, roasted	2
Olive oil, 1 tablespoon	2
Broccoli, cooked, 1 cup	2
Kiwi, 1 medium	1

FROM THE RECIPE FILE

Nuts are among the best vitamin E sources. Try the recipe for
Date Nut Balls on page 298; they're delicious, they're portable,
and they pack a good portion of the vitamin E you need every day.

Vitamin K

Vitamin K has something in common with vitamin D: both are made by
the body. Beneficial bacteria in your digestive tract produce vitamin K,
which is essential for normal blood clotting. Vitamin K is also necessary
for the growth, development, and maintenance of bones.

Although vitamin K deficiency is rare, some people are more prone
to it than others, including those with celiac disease or ulcerative coli-
tis. Certain medications, including antibiotics (for example, penicillin,
amoxicillin, and sulfamethizole) and antiseizure drugs, interfere with
vitamin K production by decreasing the bacteria in the intestinal tract
that make vitamin K. Taking high doses of aspirin on a regular basis can
interfere with the vitamin K balance in your body; so does consuming
mineral oil, cholestyramine (to control cholesterol), and quinine or qui-
nidine. Check with your doctor about vitamin K if you're taking vitamin
K–depleting medications on a long-term basis.

Daily Needs

Vitamin K requirements do not increase with pregnancy or breastfeeding;
fourteen- to eighteen-year-olds need 75 mcg daily, and women over age
nineteen need 90 mcg. Although there is no evidence for an upper-limit

requirement for vitamin K intake, there's likely no need to take vitamin K in supplement form, either.

Newborns need a boost of vitamin K because they lack adequate bacteria to make it at birth. The American Academy of Pediatrics recommends administering a one-time injection of vitamin K1 at delivery to prevent vitamin K–deficiency bleeding, a potentially life-threatening condition.

Top Food Sources

Food	Vitamin K (mcg)
Kale, 1/2 cup, cooked	531
Spinach, 1 cup, cooked	445
Spinach, 1 cup, raw	145
Broccoli, 1/2 cup, cooked	110
Asparagus, 8 spears, cooked	60
Lettuce, romaine, 1 cup, chopped	48
Peas, 1 cup, cooked	41
Blueberries, 1 cup	29
Kiwi, 1 medium	28
Soybeans, 1/2 cup, cooked	17
Cashews, 1 ounce	10

FROM THE RECIPE FILE

Broccoli Cheese Calzone (page 284) may have just a few ingredients, but it supplies some serious vitamin K as well as many other beneficial nutrients, including calcium.

B Vitamins

The B vitamins—such as B2 (riboflavin), B6, and B12—perform similar functions. In general, they are vital to helping your body derive energy from food, but each have unique jobs, too. For example, vitamin B12 is useful for building healthy blood cells; folate, also a B vitamin, helps prevent certain birth defects; and pantothenic acid (vitamin B5) is necessary for hormone production. B vitamins are found in a variety of foods.

Vitamin B1 (Thiamin)

Thiamin is notable for its role in promoting a normal nervous system and normal heart function.

Daily Needs

Nonpregnant woman, 14 to 18 years old: 1.0 mg

Nonpregnant woman, 19 to 50 years old: 1.1 mg

Pregnant, all ages: 1.4 mg

Breastfeeding, all ages: 1.5 mg

Top Food Sources

Food	Thiamin (mg)
Pork tenderloin, 3 ounces, cooked	0.8
Pecans, 1 ounce, roasted or raw	0.2
Lentils, $1/2$ cup, cooked	0.2
Long-grain white rice, enriched, $1/2$ cup, cooked	0.1
Whole-wheat bread, 1 slice (equal to 1 ounce)	0.1

Vitamin B2 (Riboflavin)

Riboflavin is necessary for energy production. It also assists the body in using the protein from the food you eat.

Daily Needs

Nonpregnant woman, 14 to 18 years old: 1.0 mg

Nonpregnant woman, 19 to 50 years old: 1.1 mg

Pregnant, all ages: 1.4 mg

Breastfeeding, all ages: 1.6 mg

Top Food Sources

Food	Riboflavin (mg)
Breakfast cereals, fortified with 100% of the Daily Value (DV) for riboflavin, 1 serving	1.7
Yogurt, plain, 1 cup	0.5
Milk, 1% low-fat, 1 cup	0.4
Almonds, 1 ounce	0.3
Cottage cheese, low-fat, $1/2$ cup	0.2
Egg, large	0.2

Niacin (Vitamin B3)

Niacin is needed for energy metabolism and for the proper growth and development of cells and tissues, particularly in the skin, central nervous system, and digestive tract.

Daily Needs

Nonpregnant woman, all ages: 14 mg

Pregnant, all ages: 18 mg

Breastfeeding, all ages: 17 mg

Top Food Sources

Food	Niacin (mg)
Chicken breast, boneless, skinless, 3 ounces, cooked	12
Turkey, light meat, 3 ounces, cooked	12
Tuna, light, canned, drained, 3 ounces	9
Salmon, Atlantic, farmed, 3 ounces, cooked	8
Beef, 95% lean, 3 ounces, cooked	5
Peanuts, 1 ounce, dry roasted	3
Lentils, $1/2$ cup, cooked	1

Pantothenic Acid (Vitamin B5)

Pantothenic acid is part of an enzyme that generates energy from food and contributes to making compounds that sustain life and support growth.

Daily Needs

Nonpregnant woman, all ages: 5 mg

Pregnant, all ages: 6 mg

Breastfeeding, all ages: 7 mg

Top Food Sources

Food	Pantothenic acid (mg)
Mushrooms, shiitake, 1 cup, cooked	5
Avocado, 1/2 whole	2
Sunflower seeds, 1 ounce, roasted	2
Yogurt, plain, 1% low-fat, 8 ounces	1
Chicken breast, boneless, skinless, 3 ounces, cooked	1
Sweet potato, medium, flesh only, baked	1

Vitamin B6

Vitamin B6 aids in protein production for new cells, bolsters the immune system, and is involved in brain development during pregnancy. It may also help the millions of women who experience nausea, vomiting, or both in the first few months of pregnancy. Consuming 100 mg or less of vitamin B6 as a dietary supplement daily may help alleviate morning sickness, but do so under the supervision of a doctor or nurse practitioner.

Daily Needs

Nonpregnant woman, 14 to 18 years old: 1.2 mg

Nonpregnant woman, 19 to 50 years old: 1.3 mg

Pregnant, all ages: 1.9 mg

Breastfeeding, all ages: 2.0 mg

Top Food Sources

Food	Vitamin B6 (mg)
Salmon, wild Atlantic, 3 ounces, cooked	0.8
Beef, top sirloin, 3 ounces, cooked	0.6
Pork tenderloin, 3 ounces, cooked	0.6
Potato, medium, flesh only, baked	0.5
Chicken breast, boneless, skinless, 3 ounces, cooked	0.5
Fortified breakfast cereals, 1 serving	about 0.5

Vitamin B12

Vitamin B12 assists in red blood cell production, helps keep the body's nerve cells healthy, and helps the body to make DNA, the genetic material in every cell of your and your baby's body.

Plant foods have no vitamin B12 unless it's added during processing. Women who eat only small amounts of animal products or who avoid them completely can become deficient in vitamin B12 unless they take supplements or eat foods with added vitamin B12. If you have celiac disease or have had gastrointestinal surgery, such as weight loss surgery, you may absorb less vitamin B12. Metformin, a drug used to treat diabetes, and medications that treat reflux disease interfere with the body's absorption and use of vitamin B12. Ask you doctor or pharmacist about the over-the-counter and prescription medications you take and how they affect your vitamin B12 needs.

Daily Needs

Nonpregnant woman, 14 to 50 years old: 2.4 mcg
Pregnant, all ages: 2.6 mcg
Breastfeeding, all ages: 2.8 mcg

Top Food Sources

Food	Vitamin B12 (mcg)
Clams, 3 ounces, cooked	84

Breakfast cereals, fortified to 100% of the Daily Value (DV), 1 serving	6
Salmon, wild Atlantic, 3 ounces, cooked	3
Haddock, 3 ounces, cooked	2
Beef, 3 ounces, cooked	2

FROM THE RECIPE FILE

Roasted Honey Orange Salmon (page 266) supplies vitamin B12
as well as choline. It's simple to make and ready in minutes.

Folate: The B-Vitamin Superstar

Folate is a B vitamin found naturally in foods. Folic acid is its synthetic cousin that is added to enriched grains and dietary supplements. Both forms of folate are worthy of attention.

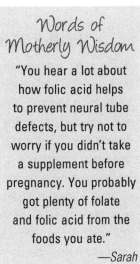

Words of Motherly Wisdom

"You hear a lot about how folic acid helps to prevent neural tube defects, but try not to worry if you didn't take a supplement before pregnancy. You probably got plenty of folate and folic acid from the foods you ate."

—*Sarah*

Folate is vital for producing new and healthy red blood cells, which are necessary for a developing baby and a healthy mother. Folate is perhaps best known for preventing neural tube defects (NTD), including spina bifida, the incomplete closure of the neural tube, which becomes baby's spinal column and brain. The neural tube develops within the first twenty-eight days of pregnancy—often before a woman suspects that she's pregnant. That's why the US Public Health Service and the CDC recommend that all women of childbearing age get the suggested folate they need every day. Half of all US pregnancies are unplanned, and consuming enough folate during early pregnancy may help to protect your baby against NTD as well as certain heart abnormalities, cleft lip, and cleft palate.

Folate is valuable throughout your entire pregnancy, too. Adequate levels of folate in the bloodstream are linked to proper growth during pregnancy as well as lower risks of anemia in the mother, miscarriage, preterm delivery, and low birth weight. Preliminary research suggests that optimal folate levels in the blood during pregnancy may protect a child from a future risk of obesity.

Women in their childbearing years (ages fourteen to fifty) who are capable of becoming pregnant should consume 400 mcg of folic acid daily from vitamin supplements, from foods fortified with folic acid, or from a combination of the two, in addition to the naturally occurring folate from foods such as legumes, 100 percent orange juice, and strawberries. Folate is not as well absorbed as folic acid. According to the Institute of Medicine, the body absorbs about 50 percent of the folate that occurs naturally in foods such as orange juice. In contrast, the body absorbs approximately 85 percent of the folic acid in fortified foods and dietary supplements, and 100 percent of the folic acid in a vitamin supplement when taken on an empty stomach.

FOR FOLIC ACID, GO FOR THE GRAIN

If you don't eat enough leafy green vegetables, legumes, or certain fruits, and if you avoid enriched grain products or skimp on them, you may not be getting the folic acid you need from food alone. Food manufacturers are required to add a certain amount of folic acid to enriched bread, cereal, flour, cornmeal, pasta, rice, and other grain products, and these products contribute a significant amount of folic acid to the diet when consumed on a regular basis. Gluten-free grain products do not always contain added folic acid, and whole grains, including breakfast cereals, may not either. All of the folate in an enriched-grain food—such as cereal, rice, bread, or pasta—is in the form of folic acid. Folic acid is listed on the food label as a percentage of the Daily Value (DV). The DV for folic acid is 400 mcg, which is how much you need every day before pregnancy. For example, if one serving of a food provides 50 percent of the DV for folic acid (that is, 200 mcg), it supplies half of your daily quota if you're not pregnant or breastfeeding, and a bit less if you are.

If you're already taking a prenatal vitamin, you don't need to take additional folic acid or another multivitamin with folic acid unless your health care provider recommends it.

Daily Needs

Nonpregnant woman, 14 to 50 years old: 400 mcg

Pregnant, all ages: 600 mcg

Breastfeeding, all ages: 500 mcg

Some women may need more folic acid, including those who are taking medications to treat type 2 diabetes, epilepsy, inflammatory bowel disease (IBD), or other conditions; women with diagnosed celiac disease; and those who drink more than one alcoholic beverage daily. Talk to your doctor about your folate requirements. If you have a family member affected by spina bifida or you have spina bifida, you should also consult your doctor before conceiving. Don't consume more than 1,000 mcg a day of folic acid unless you are advised to do so by a licensed medical professional.

Top Food Sources

Food	Folate (mcg)
Breakfast cereals fortified to 100% of the Daily Value per serving	400*
Lentils, 1/2 cup, cooked	179
White rice, enriched, 1 cup, cooked	153*
Spaghetti, enriched, 1 cup, cooked	148*
White beans, canned, drained, 1/2 cup	123
Broccoli, 1 cup, cooked	103
Orange juice, 8 ounces	74
Spinach, 1 cup, raw	58
Strawberries, sliced, 1 cup	40
Bread, enriched, 2 slices	26*

*Contains folic acid, the synthetic form of folate that is added to grains and dietary supplements.

Choline

You may not know much about choline; it's one of those nutrients that doesn't generate a lot of buzz. Yet choline is necessary for the normal functioning of all cells, especially those in the liver and the central nervous system, which includes the brain. Some observational research suggests that choline works with folic acid to help reduce the risk for NTD.

Animal studies show that choline is critical for brain development, particularly of the hippocampus, the brain's so-called memory center. The hippocampus is one of the only areas in the brain that continues to produce nerve cells throughout life. During pregnancy, the baby's organ growth, particularly the growth of the brain, happens quickly, and the mother's diet must supply the choline that the developing child requires.

Evidence suggests that many women are low in choline before they conceive. Choline can be made by the body in small amounts, but you must get nearly all you need from food. Don't rely on multivitamin pills or prenatal supplements to meet choline needs. Most dietary supplements supply little or no choline. Choline is widely available in the food supply. High-protein foods have the most choline.

Daily Needs

Nonpregnant woman, 14 to 50 years old: 425 mg

Pregnant, all ages: 450 mg

Breastfeeding, all ages: 550 mg

Do not consume more than 3,500 mg of choline daily.

Top Food Sources

Food	Choline (mg)
Egg, whole, large	125
Pork tenderloin, 3 ounces, cooked	103
Ground beef, 3 ounces, cooked	85
Cod, Atlantic, 3 ounces, cooked	84
Shrimp, 3 ounces, cooked	81
Chicken breast, boneless, skinless, 3 ounces, cooked	78

Salmon, sockeye, 3 ounces, cooked	65
Broccoli, cooked, 1 cup	64
Soybeans, $1/4$ cup, roasted	53
Garbanzo beans, $1/2$ cup, cooked	35
Peanut butter, 2 tablespoons	20

Vitamin C

Vitamin C is best known for its role in building and maintaining a strong immune system that fights infection, defends cells against damage, and helps to ward off cancer. Vitamin C also supports healthy bones, teeth, and connective tissue; keeps blood vessels strong and resilient; and promotes healthy red blood cells. Vitamin C improves the body's uptake of iron from plant foods, such as spinach, legumes (beans), and iron-fortified grains, including cereal, bread, and pasta.

Daily Needs

Nonpregnant woman, 14 to 18 years old: 65 mg

Nonpregnant woman, 19 to 50 years old: 75 mg

Pregnant, 14 to 18 years old: 80 mg

Pregnant, 19 to 50 years old: 85 mg

Breastfeeding, 14 to 18 years old: 115 mg

Breastfeeding, 19 to 50 years old: 120 mg

Smokers need 35 milligrams of additional vitamin C daily, in part because cigarette smoke increases the amount of vitamin C the body requires to repair cell damage caused by free radicals (unstable oxygen compounds in the blood created by smoking). Secondhand smoke increases vitamin C requirements, too, but there are no recommendations for intake for those exposed to secondhand smoke on a regular basis.

Do not consume more than 1,800 mg a day of vitamin C if you are fourteen to eighteen years old and are pregnant or nursing, and no more than 2,000 mg a day if you are nineteen or older and are pregnant or nursing.

Top Food Sources

Food	Vitamin C (mg)
Orange juice, 8 ounces	124
Broccoli, 1 cup, cooked	101
Strawberries, sliced, 1 cup	98
Red bell pepper, sliced, 1 cup, raw	74
Orange, 1 medium	64
Raspberries, 1 cup	32
Potato, medium, baked	22
Tomato, 1 medium	17

MINERALS

Minerals are part of every process that supports life in your body and in your baby's body. Minerals are involved in the normal functioning of the muscles and the nervous system and in bolstering the immune system. They also provide structural support, as part of the bones, teeth, and red blood cells. Your body doesn't make minerals, so you need to get them from food, from dietary supplements, or from a combination of the two.

Iron

Iron is vital to the production of hemoglobin, the part of red blood cells that transports oxygen to the cells in your body and your child's body. It's also part of myoglobin, which supplies oxygen to your muscles. Iron plays a role in building a strong immune system, in energy production, in ensuring a healthy birth weight, and in the proper development of a child's brain and nervous system.

There's a surge in red blood cell production during pregnancy to meet your growing baby's need for oxygen, so it's easy to see why pregnancy dramatically increases iron needs. Your body can store iron, which is why heading into pregnancy with adequate iron reserves helps prevent iron-deficiency anemia, the most common nutritional deficit in the world, during pregnancy. Your body can tap into its stored iron when your intake is below what it should be, but problems may arise when your iron intake is low for a prolonged time. When there's not enough iron to go around, the red blood cells take priority, and that comes at the expense of brain and other tissues that need iron.

IRON ON BOARD

Most babies are born with a six-month supply of iron, but some have less at birth because babies accumulate most of their iron stores toward the last part of pregnancy. Preterm infants (babies who did not develop fully in the womb because they were born too early) and children born to women with diabetes are prone to iron deficiency because they have lower iron reserves at birth.

With the exception of the iron contained in eggs, the iron in food is one of two types: heme or nonheme iron. (Egg iron is about half of each type). Heme iron is the most common form in animal foods, including meat, seafood, and poultry. Red meat and dark white meat, such as dark chicken meat, contain more iron than white meat. Nonheme iron is the only form of iron in plant foods and in fortified products, such as bread, cereal, pasta, and rice. The body absorbs heme iron better than it absorbs nonheme iron.

You can significantly improve your body's uptake of iron by pairing foods high in vitamin C with foods containing nonheme iron. For instance, combine the following: white bean soup with kale; black bean burger with tomatoes; orange juice and iron-fortified breakfast cereal; strawberries and a sandwich made with fortified bread; iron-enriched pasta and tomato sauce; burgers (ground turkey or beef) on iron-enriched rolls with a slice of tomato.

Daily Needs

Nonpregnant woman, 14 to 18 years old: 15 mg

Nonpregnant woman, 19 to 50 years old: 18 mg

Pregnant, all ages: 27 mg

**Breastfeeding (if periods have resumed),
14 to 50 years old:** 18 mg

**Breastfeeding (if periods have not resumed),
14 to 18 years old:** 10 mg

**Breastfeeding (if periods have not resumed),
19 to 50 years old:** 9 mg

Top Food Sources

Food	Iron (mg)
Breakfast cereals fortified with 100% of the Daily Value for iron, 1 serving	18
Oysters, eastern, 3 ounces, cooked	8
Spinach, 1 cup, cooked	6
Oatmeal, enriched, instant, 1 packet	4
White beans, canned, drained, 1/2 cup	4
Rice, white, enriched, 1 cup, cooked	3
Beef, 95% lean, ground, cooked, 3 ounces	2
Soybeans, 1/2 cup, cooked	2
Tofu, 1/4 block	2

FROM THE RECIPE FILE

Beef is a source of iron and zinc, two nutrients you need every day, whether or not you're pregnant or breastfeeding. See page 290 for a recipe for Slow-Cooker Beef and Mushroom Stew.

Zinc

Zinc is an all-around nutrient. Zinc helps to produce DNA, the genetic material that is the blueprint for every new cell in your body and your baby's body. It is also involved in energy production and is necessary for brain development. Zinc is part of insulin, the hormone that regulates blood glucose levels, and it contributes to a healthy immune system and wound healing. These are just some of the ways that zinc supports good health.

Zinc is particularly abundant in animal foods, including meat and certain seafood. Many breakfast cereals are fortified with zinc. Because zinc is primarily found in the germ and bran portions of grains, milling—a process used to make refined grains, such as that contained in white bread and crackers—removes a large portion of natural zinc from these grains.

Vegetarians and vegans may require as much as 50 percent more zinc than meat eaters because of certain elements in plant foods that impair zinc uptake by the body. If you avoid animal products or eat very few on a regular basis, be sure to choose whole grains (like brown rice or whole-wheat bread) and fortified grains as part of a balanced diet, and take a multivitamin/multimineral pill with 100 percent of the Daily Value for zinc before, during, and after pregnancy.

Daily Needs
Nonpregnant woman, 14 to 18 years old: 9 mg

Nonpregnant woman, 19 to 50 years old: 8 mg

Pregnant, 14 to 18 years old: 12 mg

Pregnant, 19 to 50 years old: 11 mg

Breastfeeding, 14 to 18 years old: 13 mg

Breastfeeding, 19 to 50 years old: 12 mg

Do not consume more than 40 mg of zinc a day from supplements.

Top Food Sources

Food	Zinc (mg)
Oysters, eastern, 3 ounces, cooked	67
Crab, Alaska king, 3 ounces, cooked	6
Beef, ground, 95% lean, 3 ounces, cooked	5
Turkey, skinless, dark meat, 3 ounces, cooked	3
Pork tenderloin, 3 ounces, cooked	3
Yogurt, plain, fat-free, 1 cup	2
Wheat germ, 2 tablespoons	2

Calcium

Calcium is the most abundant mineral in the human body. It plays a central part in the function of nearly every cell, in addition to its best-known role of building and maintaining strong bones and teeth. Although your skeleton stores nearly all of the calcium in your body, about one percent of the body's calcium resides in the blood and the tissues, perpetuating life by promoting normal muscle contraction, nerve transmission, and a regular heartbeat.

> ### Words of Motherly Wisdom
>
> "As a vegan, I don't drink milk or eat dairy products, but I do make sure I get the calcium I need from a variety of calcium-added foods and plant foods that naturally contain calcium, too."
>
> —Dina

Bones act as your calcium "bank account." When you don't get enough calcium in your diet, the body withdraws the mineral from your bones to keep blood calcium concentration within a healthy range. During pregnancy, a woman's body becomes highly efficient at absorbing calcium, which is why calcium needs don't change after you conceive. However, most women enter pregnancy consuming considerably less calcium than they require, and only a small percentage of women in their child-bearing years get the calcium they need every day.

Dairy foods are naturally rich in calcium. Women who completely avoid dairy foods or who eat them sparingly should consider adding more calcium-fortified foods to their eating pattern. Multivitamin/mineral pills and prescription and over-the-counter prenatal supplements contain far less calcium than individual calcium supplements. Try to meet your calcium needs with food or with a combination of food and calcium supplements, if necessary.

Daily Needs

Nonpregnant woman, 14 to 18 years old: 1,300 mg

Nonpregnant woman, 19 to 50 years old: 1,000 mg

Pregnant, 14 to 18 years old: 1,300 mg

Pregnant, 19 to 50 years old: 1,000 mg

Breastfeeding, 14 to 18 years old: 1,300 mg

Breastfeeding, 19 to 50 years old: 1,000 mg

If you're 19 to 50 years old, do not consume more than 2,500 mg of calcium on a daily basis, and no more than 3,000 mg daily if you're 14 to 18 years old.

REALITY CHECK: LACTOSE INTOLERANCE

You have lactose intolerance. You love dairy but it doesn't love you back. Try lactose-free milk, yogurt, and cottage cheese, which are very low in lactose or 100 percent lactose-free. You can also take lactase pills or enzymes (with food) to break down lactose. Almond milk and soy milk are often fortified with calcium and other essential nutrients and are beneficial for those with lactose intolerance.

Top Food Sources

Use the list below to help you to include enough calcium every day. If you don't typically get enough calcium from foods, see the sidebar "The Best Calcium Supplements" for which supplements to take.

Food	Calcium (mg)
Tofu, firm, prepared with calcium sulfate, $1/4$ block	553
Yogurt, plain, fat-free, 1 cup	452
Soy milk, fortified, Silk brand Original	450
Orange juice, calcium-added, 8 ounces	364
Yogurt, fruit-flavored, low-fat, 1 cup	345
Milk, plain, 1 cup	305
Milk, lactose-free, 1 cup	300
Cheddar cheese, 1 ounce	201
Cottage cheese, 2% reduced-fat, $1/2$ cup	125
Ice cream, vanilla, 1 cup	84
Broccoli, 1 cup, cooked	62

THE BEST CALCIUM SUPPLEMENTS

It's not only how much calcium you consume; it's the quality that matters, too. Dietary supplements that contain calcium carbonate (including some antacids) and calcium citrate are highly favorable because the body absorbs calcium carbonate and calcium citrate better than other forms of calcium. Calcium citrate malate (CCM) is a form of calcium that is used to fortify certain juices. Choose juices with CCM; it's absorbed well by the body. Don't take more than 500 mg of supplemental calcium at a time; separating calcium doses promotes peak absorption.

Stealthy Tips for Getting More Dairy in Your Diet

Here's how to include more milk and other dairy foods in a balanced eating plan:

- Stir ricotta cheese or pureed cottage cheese into warm or cold pasta dishes.

- Make a fruit smoothie with yogurt or milk.

- Enjoy hot chocolate or chocolate milk made with low-fat or fat-free milk.

- Make mashed potatoes with evaporated milk instead of regular milk. Evaporated milk supplies twice the calcium.

- Prepare condensed soups with low-fat or fat-free milk instead of water.

- Make oatmeal in the microwave with milk instead of water.

FROM THE RECIPE FILE

Strawberry Peach Sipper (page 229) features a cup of fruit and
a cup of dairy. Fortified soy milk, typically rich in added calcium, counts
as a dairy food. Calcium levels vary, so look for brands with at least
30 percent of the Daily Value for calcium listed on the food label.

Magnesium

Every cell in your body and your baby's needs magnesium. Magnesium helps to regulate muscle and nerve function, keeps the heart rhythm steady, and bolsters immunity. It's also important for promoting normal blood pressure and boosting bone strength. Magnesium is involved in energy metabolism and protein production, too.

Daily Needs

Nonpregnant woman, 14 to 18 years old: 360 mg

Nonpregnant woman, 19 to 30 years old: 310 mg

Nonpregnant woman, 31 to 50 years old: 320 mg

Pregnant, 14 to 18 years old: 400 mg

Pregnant, 19 to 50 years old: 350 mg

Pregnant, 31 to 50 years: 360 mg

Breastfeeding, 14 to 18 years old: 360 mg

Breastfeeding, 19 to 30 years old: 310 mg

Breastfeeding, 31 to 50 years: 320 mg

Magnesium is found primarily in plant foods. If you don't eat at least five servings of a variety of fruits and vegetables every day (including legumes, which are vegetables) you may be missing out on magnesium.

There is no recommended upper limit for magnesium from food. However, do not consume more than 350 mg of magnesium from dietary supplements or medications. For example, laxatives may contain magnesium. Large doses of magnesium can cause diarrhea and abdominal cramping. To be sure you're not overdoing magnesium, ask your health care provider about all over-the-counter and prescription medications you take when you're pregnant and breastfeeding.

Top Food Sources

Food	Magnesium (mg)
Soybeans, 1/2 cup, roasted	125
Spinach, 1 cup, cooked	87

Brown rice, long-grain, 1 cup, cooked	79
Almonds, 1 ounce, roasted	77
Cashews, 1 ounce, roasted	74
Black beans, canned, $1/2$ cup	60
Peanuts, 1 ounce, roasted	50
Whole-wheat bread, 2 slices	48
Potato, 1 medium, flesh only, baked	39
Lentils, $1/2$ cup, cooked	35
Broccoli, 1 cup, cooked	32
Banana, 1 medium	32
Milk, 1% low-fat, 8 ounces	27
Orange juice, 8 ounces	27
Halibut, 3 ounces, cooked	24

FROM THE RECIPE FILE

Beans are a convenient way to include more magnesium.
This Taco Salad (page 272) supplies nearly 40 percent of
your daily magnesium needs, and it tastes great, too!

Sodium

You might think of sodium as a villain because of its role in high blood pressure and bloating. True, sodium helps your body to retain fluid, which can cause swelling as well as elevated blood pressure. However, sodium's role in retaining water is also beneficial. That's because your body, and your baby's body, is made up mostly of water that you want to keep for many reasons.

Maintaining a normal fluid balance is critical to a healthy blood pressure, no matter what your life stage. Even though sodium is often criticized, it is necessary for normal muscle contraction and nerve function. Sodium also transports nutrients into cells and carries waste products for removal from the body.

Sodium is a component of nearly every food, so you can't completely avoid it, nor should you, but you can limit its intake. Fresh foods are relatively low in sodium, whereas highly processed fare—such as fast foods, take-out and restaurant fare, canned soups and vegetables, and frozen dinners—have more. Most of the sodium we consume is found in processed and premade foods. Processed foods can be high in added salt (sodium chloride), and they often also include sodium-containing additives such as monosodium glutamate (MSG), sodium citrate, and disodium phosphate.

> ### Words of Motherly Wisdom
>
> "I never realized how much sodium was in the foods I ate on a daily basis until I started reading food labels. Now I go for lower-sodium versions whenever I can."
>
> —Shana

Daily Needs

All adults should limit sodium intake to less than 2,300 mg a day, according to the 2015–2020 Dietary Guidelines for Americans. If you have high blood pressure, reducing your sodium intake can help to lower it. However, there's no reason to eat less than about 2,300 milligrams of sodium a day during pregnancy unless you are advised to do so for health reasons.

Check out the list below for sources of sodium in common foods.

Top Food Sources

Food	Sodium (mg)
Salt, 1 teaspoon	2,300
Grilled chicken sandwich, fast-food	1,237
Soy sauce, 1 tablespoon	1,024
Cottage cheese, 1% low-fat, 1 cup	918
Pizza, 4 ounces, frozen	890
Soup, canned, 1 cup	700–1,200
Vegetable juice, canned, 8 ounces	653
Corn, canned, drained, 1 cup	571

Potassium

Potassium is essential for the body's growth and supports good health in many ways. It works with sodium to promote fluid balance. Potassium also plays an essential role in nerve cell function and in proper muscle contraction. Cellular enzymes require potassium to work properly, and muscles need potassium to store carbohydrates to use as energy. Potassium helps to strengthen and maintain bones by counteracting calcium losses from the body caused by high-sodium diets.

You may think that orange juice and bananas are the only good potassium sources. However, fresh and lightly processed foods from all the food groups provide significant amounts of potassium, too. Unless you're told otherwise by your doctor, aim for 4,700 mg of potassium daily.

Top Food Sources

Food	Potassium (mg)
Potato, medium, with skin, baked	941
Carrot juice, 1 cup	689
White beans, canned, drained, 1/2 cup	595
Butternut squash, cubed, 1 cup, cooked	582
Yogurt, plain, fat-free, 1 cup	579
Sweet potato, medium, with skin, baked	542
Salmon, Atlantic, wild, 3 ounces, cooked	534
Orange juice, fresh, 8 ounces	496
Great Northern beans, canned, 1/2 cup	460
Broccoli, chopped, 1 cup, cooked	458
Halibut, 3 ounces, cooked	449
Soybeans, mature, 1/2 cup, cooked	443
Cantaloupe, cubed, 1 cup	427
Banana, 1 medium	422
Chocolate milk, 8 ounces	418–425
Pork tenderloin, 3 ounces, cooked	383
Milk, fat-free, 8 ounces	382

Dried apricots, $^1/_4$ cup	378
Lentils, cooked, $^1/_2$ cup	366
Avocado, $^1/_2$ cup	364
Raisins, $^1/_4$ cup	272
Chicken breast, boneless, skinless, 3 ounces, cooked	218

FROM THE RECIPE FILE

Creamy Sweet Potato Soup (page 287) is packed with potassium—
and several other vitamins and minerals, too.

Iodine

Iodine is a major component of the thyroid hormones that regulate a number of key processes in your body and in your baby's. During pregnancy, thyroxine and other thyroid hormones are necessary for the myelination of the nerves in your baby's body. Myelination is the process that ensures speedy and correct communication among the nerve cells and in the brain.

You need adequate iodine intake to insure that your baby's brain develops to its fullest potential. Severe iodine deficiency in mom can lead to serious effects for her baby, including mental retardation, but even moderately insufficient intake may take a subtle toll on a child's brain. Many people get enough iodine, yet US women in their childbearing years are among those most likely to consume inadequate amounts of iodine.

Daily Needs

The Institute of Medicine (IOM) recommends the following iodine intakes for women of childbearing age:

Nonpregnant woman, 14 to 50 years old: 150 mcg

Pregnant, all ages: 220 mcg

Breastfeeding, all ages: 290 mcg

Limits of daily intake, nonpregnant, pregnant, and breast-feeding: 14 to 18 years old, 900 mcg; 19 to 50 years old, 1,100 mcg

Mom's intake of adequate amounts of iodine is important for baby's brain starting at about the tenth week of pregnancy and throughout breastfeeding. Certain foods are better sources of the mineral than others, but levels can vary. Seafood and sea vegetables, such as kelp, nori, kombu, and wakame, are reliable iodine sources. Fruits and vegetables contain iodine, but the amount varies depending on the iodine content of the soil and other factors.

It's difficult to identify packaged foods with iodine because iodine content is not listed in the Nutrition Facts label. Eat the suggested 8 to 12 ounces of seafood weekly as part of a balanced diet to help satisfy iodine needs. You don't need to avoid salt, and when you use it at home, make sure it's iodized, as iodized salt has added iodine.

It's not always easy to fulfill your daily iodine quota with food. The American Thyroid Association (ATA) recommends that pregnant and breastfeeding women and women who are planning to become pregnant consume at least 250 micrograms (mcg) of iodine daily, which is slightly more than the 220 mcg recommended by the IOM. To insure that you meet your need for iodine, the ATA recommends that pregnant and breastfeeding women take 150 mcg of iodine as a dietary supplement every day to fill in iodine gaps. Choose a multivitamin with potassium iodide, as this form of iodine is well absorbed by the body. Many over-the-counter multivitamins contain 150 mcg of iodine.

Top Food Sources

Food	Iodine (mcg)
Seaweed, whole or sheet, 1 gram	16–2,984
Cod, 3 ounces, baked	99
Yogurt, plain, low-fat, 1 cup	75
Iodized salt, 1/4 teaspoon	71
Milk, 2% reduced-fat, 8 ounces	56
Pasta, enriched, 1 cup, cooked	27
Tuna, canned, drained, 3 ounces	17

PHYTONUTRIENTS

Ellagic acid, phenethyl isothiocyanate, lutein, zeaxanthin, and sulfora-phane—this sounds like a mess of chemicals you'd find in the most processed of foods. However, these compounds, collectively known as *phytochemicals* or *phytonutrients,* are naturally occurring substances in plants, such as raspberries, carrots, and cauliflower. Phytonutrients are credited for providing a multitude of health benefits, including reducing the inflammation that may give rise to heart disease and cancer, boosting immunity, and improving eyesight.

Many phytonutrients serve more than one purpose. Some provide pigments that brighten fruits and vegetables, including blueberries, watermelon, and cantaloupe. Others repel damage to their host plants from germs or strong sunlight. Still other phytonutrients, such as beta-carotene, serve as the raw material for vitamin A in the body. Beta-carotene is one of the phytonutrients that helps to head off cell damage that could threaten your health and your child's development.

Nobody knows exactly how many beneficial substances plant foods supply, but it's probably in the thousands. Brightly colored fruits and vegetables, such as tomatoes, broccoli, oranges, spinach, and sweet potatoes, are among the foods richest in phytonutrients, but white produce, such as mushrooms, cauliflower, and bananas are also good sources of substances that support health. Whole grains supply phy-tonutrients, too. Plant-based eating plans provide a steady supply of phytonutrients.

NOW YOU KNOW

You've finished reading this chapter, and you've learned a lot. You know that some fats are better than others, that you don't have to drink plain water to satisfy fluid needs, what the latest research says about caffeine before and during pregnancy, and much more. Don't worry if you don't recall everything you've read; you know where to find the information when you need it.

The next chapter takes you another step in your pregnancy journey.

You'll be leaving behind the details about specific nutrients and learning how to put together a personalized eating plan that's right for you with delicious and healthy foods. Chapter 3 is all about MyPlate, a balanced approach to healthy eating that nearly everyone can easily follow, and, even better, enjoy.

3

MyPlate Plans: What to Eat Before, During, and After Pregnancy

Chapter 2 covered the specific nutrients you and your baby need to support good health. It's great to understand why and how to get the energy-producing nutrients (carbohydrates, fat, and protein) you need, as well as how to meet your requirements for vitamins and minerals, but now it's time to translate that knowledge into what to eat every day. This chapter is about designing a balanced, varied, and enjoyable eating plan that's right for you.

STEP UP TO MYPLATE

MyPlate is an eating program designed to help make it easier to plan and enjoy a balanced diet. MyPlate is meant for most healthy people ages two and older, including pregnant women and breastfeeding women with uncomplicated pregnancies. In its simplest form, MyPlate shows you what to actually put on your plate and in your glass. MyPlate also guides you to make the best choices from each food group at every meal.

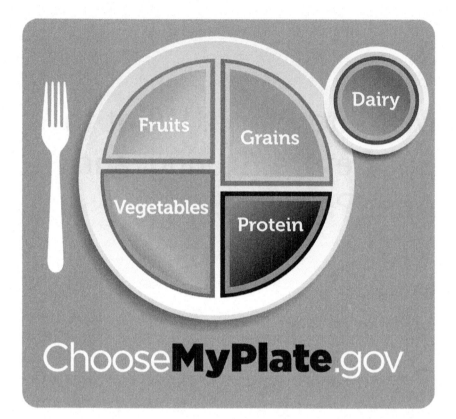

There's no single healthy way to eat, but there are better food choices to make no matter what your eating style. MyPlate is about more than how much to eat from each of the five foods groups (grains, vegetables, fruits, milk, and protein); it explains why you need those foods. MyPlate's recommendations are based on the Dietary Guidelines for Americans, which were developed by the US Department of Health and Human Services and the US Department of Agriculture.

Balance, variety, and moderation rule MyPlate, which also includes physical activity recommendations. The best part of MyPlate is that it can be personalized, whether you eat meat; follow a vegetarian plan but include milk, seafood, and/or eggs; are vegan; or gluten-free.

FIGURE YOUR CALORIE NEEDS

How will you know how much to eat from each of MyPlate's food groups? You'll need to figure out a suggested daily calorie intake based on your age, gender, and whether you're pregnant or breastfeeding. Physical activity level is also part of the calorie equation. Use the following guidelines to determine your activity level.

If you exercise . . .	Then you're . . .
Less than 30 minutes on most days	Sedentary
30 to 60 minutes on most days	Moderately active
60 to 90 minutes on most days	Active

It's tempting to regard exercise as just a weight-loss method or even as punishment, but it's more than that. Walking, biking, swimming, hiking, and other aerobic activities strengthen your heart, lower your blood pressure, and reduce risk for certain cancers. Physical activity enhances weight-loss efforts, particularly when combined with eating fewer calories, and exercise is also good for your overall health. The Physical Activity Guidelines for Americans suggest that most healthy adults get a minimum of thirty minutes a day of moderate-intensity exercise, such as brisk walking. The guidelines for exercise during pregnancy are discussed in chapter 4.

Start increasing your physical activity on a regular basis to reap the many benefits (see chapter 1). Try to fit in at least thirty minutes of moderate-intensity activity on most days of the week. Let your health care provider know that you're embarking on a healthier eating regime and exercise routine to get in better shape before you conceive, or during pregnancy, especially if you have a medical condition.

Now that know your physical activity level, you can estimate the number of daily calories that's best for you. The calorie levels in the chart below from the Dietary Guidelines serve as suggestions to promote weight maintenance in men and in women who are not pregnant, or who are in their first trimester (less than thirteen weeks pregnant).

REALITY CHECK: DO YOU MOVE ENOUGH?

Every move you make uses calories. However, you may be overestimating the calories you burn. Assuming that you use more energy than you do may backfire, because you might eat more than you should based on your perceived physical activity. Overeating for your activity level can result in weight gain with time, and may lead to frustration when you increase activity but the pounds won't come off. Some physical activities are better than others. For example, a thirty-minute brisk walk every day burns more calories than getting up off the couch ten times to change the television channel, and it offers more health benefits, too. Even so, getting up to change the channel is better than using the remote while lounging on the couch, because any movement is better than none.

DAILY CALORIE NEEDS

Age (years)	Sedentary	Moderately Active	Active
		WOMEN	
14–18	1,800	2,000	2,400
19–25	2,000	2,200	2,400
26–30	1,800	2,000	2,400
31–50	1,800	2,000	2,200
		MEN	
16–18	2,400	2,800	3,200
19–20	2,600	2,800	3,000
21–35	2,400	2,800	3,000
36–40	2,400	2,600	2,800
41–55	2,200	2,400	2,800

THE MYPLATE PREPREGNANCY PLAN

You have just one more decision to make before you finalize your daily calorie budget. If you're not pregnant, would you like to lose or gain weight to help you achieve a weight within the healthy weight range, or would you like to stay your same weight?

For more help, see the information about body mass index (BMI) in chapter 1, if you haven't read about it already. BMI serves as a guideline for deciding if you should lose weight, gain weight, or maintain your weight before trying for a baby. If you are more than thirteen weeks pregnant, choose a calorie level (it will be your prepregnancy daily calorie intake) from the chart above and skip to the MyPlate Pregnancy Plan for more guidance about your calorie needs during the second and third trimesters. If you're breastfeeding, choose a daily prepregnancy level from the chart and see the MyPlate Postpregnancy Plan for more information about suggested calorie intake.

As discussed in chapter 1, starting pregnancy at a healthy weight is important to your child's growth and development, and to your health, too. Losing weight prior to pregnancy isn't just for women, however. Get your partner involved in a lifestyle that incorporates nutritious foods and regular physical activity. Healthy habits benefit both of you, and may improve your fertility as a couple. Developing better eating habits before you have a baby might make it easier to put healthy meals and snacks together later on, when life gets busier.

You may be eager to drop some pounds and get on with starting a family, but you must allow a reasonable amount of time to lose weight. Cutting calories, increasing physical activity, or doing both will likely help you to shed pounds. A two-pound weekly weight loss (or less) is considered safest. Losing weight isn't an exact science, but it's generally thought that if you want to lose about a pound a week, you should try to achieve a 500-calorie-a-day deficit by eating less, moving around more, or both. For example, you could cut your daily calorie intake by 250 and burn 250 calories more every day in physical activity to achieve the 500-calorie-a-day deficit.

Very-low-calorie diets (under 1,600 calories a day) may speed up weight loss, but they make it very difficult for you to get the nutrients— including protein, fiber, and folate—that are necessary to prime your body for pregnancy. Furthermore, it's difficult to stick with lower-calorie eating programs in the long run. Instead of cheating yourself of good nutrition and eating satisfaction, use the time before pregnancy as an opportunity to build a better diet that benefits you and your future child. Losing weight does not mean dietary deprivation. Even small subtractions on a regular basis, such as skipping a sugary granola bar, a handful of candy, or snack chips can add up to better weight control.

To gain weight, add 250 to 500 calories a day to your calorie budget (for example, half a turkey sandwich and a glass of low-fat milk), or even more if you increase your physical activity. Keep track of what you're taking in, and be sure it measures up to what your MyPlate plan suggests. You could be satisfying your daily calorie needs but underestimating your physical activity, so you would require more food to put on the pounds. If you're not able to gain weight easily, seek help from a registered dietitian nutritionist (RDN).

REALITY CHECK: WEIGHT LOSS MATH

Calorie calculations are guidelines for shedding or gaining pounds, and they do not guarantee exact results. Everyone's body reacts differently to weight-loss or weight-gain efforts, but eating nutritious foods most of the time and getting adequate exercise are steps in the right direction, no matter what it says on the scale.

THE MYPLATE PREGNANCY PLAN

This may come as surprise, but even when you're pregnant you don't need to eat more right away. During the first trimester (the first thirteen weeks of pregnancy), continue to follow your MyPlate Prepregnancy Plan, described in this chapter. However, if you were trying to lose weight prior to conception, stop now that you're expecting a child. Add back the calories you cut from your diet for weight loss, and use a calorie level that will help you maintain your prepregnancy weight. You may not have reached your weight-loss goal, but pregnancy is no time to diet, and doing so could be potentially harmful to your baby. Even if you don't reach your goal weight before conceiving, having shed some pounds has moved you closer to the healthy weight range, and that's an accomplishment for you and your future child.

A full-term (forty-week) pregnancy requires tens of thousands of calories of energy. Although you may feel hungrier at times and experience more food cravings during the first weeks of pregnancy, your calorie needs won't increase until the end of the first trimester (at fourteen weeks). That makes sense, given that after the initial thirteen weeks of pregnancy, your baby is only about as big as your thumb. The baby's size doesn't diminish the importance of a balanced diet, however. You still need to eat healthy foods, get 600 micrograms of folic acid every day, and avoid substances, such as alcohol, that harm a developing child. You need to eat healthy to keep up your strength for what's ahead!

> *Words of*
> *Motherly Wisdom*
>
> "Having an eating plan to go by is definitely a plus, but you don't have to adhere to it 100 percent of the time to get good results."
> —*Sarah*

A child begins growing in earnest at the start of the second trimester. Once you've passed the thirteenth week, your daily calorie budget increases by about 350. In the third trimester, you need about 450 more calories every day than you did in the first trimester and when you were not pregnant.

Perhaps you envision spending your new, higher-calorie windfall on brownie sundaes or a huge pile of nachos with cheese, but that's not a good idea on a regular basis. Adding food isn't enough during pregnancy—it needs to count for you and your baby. Make the most of the extra food you eat by including nutrient-rich choices most of the time. Of course, you can still indulge in your favorite foods, just not every day.

Below is a list with some ways to add extra pregnancy calories with nutrient-rich foods that taste great and are good for you and your baby. The following combinations contain about 350 calories each. You can add them to your pregnancy diet in these combinations or separately:

- 1 cup of whole-grain cereal with 8 ounces of 1% low-fat milk and half a medium banana

- 8 ounces of vanilla low-fat yogurt mixed with 1 ounce of slivered almonds

- A medium pear with 1½ ounces of reduced-fat cheese and six whole-grain crackers

- A medium apple smeared with 2 tablespoons of peanut butter, almond butter, or sunflower seed butter, along with 8 ounces of 1% low-fat milk

- Two hard-cooked eggs and half a whole-grain bagel with 1 teaspoon of trans fat–free (nonhydrogenated) tub margarine or butter and 1 teaspoon of jam

The following choices provide about 450 calories each for when the third trimester comes around:

- A mini whole-grain bagel topped with $1/2$ cup of low-fat cottage cheese, and 8 ounces of low-sodium vegetable juice

- A nut-butter and banana sandwich: two slices of whole-wheat bread, two tablespoons of peanut butter, almond butter, or sunflower seed butter, and half a large banana or two tablespoons of raisins

- 3 ounces of roasted chicken, one medium baked sweet potato with 2 teaspoons of trans fat–free (nonhydrogenated) tub margarine or butter, 8 ounces of 1% low-fat chocolate milk or hot cocoa

- 4 ounces of cooked lean beef and two slices of whole-grain bread

- A fruit smoothie made with 1 cup of 1% low-fat milk, 1 cup of fresh or frozen berries, and 1 teaspoon of sugar (if desired), with a 2-ounce whole-grain bagel and 2 teaspoons of trans fat–free (nonhydrogenated) tub margarine or butter

DOUBLY BLESSED: TWIN PREGNANCY NUTRITION

It makes sense that a twin pregnancy requires more calories (and protein, as discussed in chapter 2). Your daily calorie needs for twins are based on your prepregnancy weight. Here are three examples of calorie estimates for a twin pregnancy based on a woman who is five feet five inches tall:

Underweight (113 pounds): About 2,100–2,600 calories per day

Normal weight (135 pounds): 2,400–2,800 calories per day

Overweight (162 pounds): 2,200–2,600 calories per day

These calculations provide a guideline for how many calories to eat for twins, but it's probably best to make an appointment with an RDN for a tailor-made eating plan.

THE MYPLATE POSTPREGNANCY PLAN

You've had your baby and you'd like your prebaby body back. That's reasonable, but it probably won't happen quickly. Don't be taken in by all the headlines about celebrities who can fit into their prepregnancy clothes six weeks after delivery; they are exceptions to the rule. For most women, regaining their before-baby fitness is a slow and steady process that can take several months to a year. If you're not breastfeeding, refer to the MyPlate Prepregnancy Plan to guide you back to a healthy eating regimen.

During the first six months, breastfeeding women require almost as many calories as during the second trimester of pregnancy: 330 calories a day more than their prepregnancy needs. After six months, you need about 400 extra calories each day, or close to the amount you needed during the third trimester. The actual calorie cost of producing milk to nourish a child is more than 330 or 400 calories a day, but the body mobilizes some of the energy stored in the body fat you gained during pregnancy to make breast milk.

Words of
Motherly Wisdom

"When I found out I was pregnant the first time, it was a bit of an eating free-for-all at first! But I managed to get on track and ate right the rest of my pregnancy."
—Deb

Whether you're breastfeeding or not, don't attempt weight loss until six weeks after delivery day, and when you do, take a moderate approach when curbing calorie intake. Your body needs time to recover from pregnancy and childbirth, and you need all the strength and energy you can muster to care for a newborn. Shortchanging your diet right after delivery is no good for you or your family.

WHEN YOU NEED MORE HELP: ASK A REGISTERED DIETITIAN NUTRITIONIST

MyPlate serves as an excellent foundation for healthy eating, but you may need more assistance with your food plan because of a chronic condition, such as diabetes, disordered eating, or high blood pressure, or because you're having more than one baby. Perhaps you just want more information. In any case, consult a registered dietitian nutritionist (RDN). RDNs have a minimum of a bachelor's degree from an accredited college or university, and they've also completed an accredited supervised practice experience, such as a twelve-month dietetic internship at a hospital. Many RDNs hold advanced degrees. RDNs are trained to tailor an eating plan to your needs, accounting for your medical history, health goals, and life stage. For a free referral to an RDN in your area, go to www.eatright.org/find-an-expert.

PUTTING IT ALL TOGETHER: THE MYPLATE PLANS

To build a balanced eating plan, keep in mind the number and the size of the servings to select from each food group in MyPlate. To find out how many servings are right for you, locate the calorie level you estimated earlier based on your age and activity level, then pick a pattern from the chart below. If you're in the first trimester, you don't need extra calories yet. Most pregnant women need between 2,200 and 2,900 calories daily during the second and third trimesters, and breastfeeding women may need more. The plans for the 1,600-, 1,800-, and 2,000-calorie levels are not meant for pregnant or breastfeeding women. The 1600-calorie level is most appropriate for sedentary women who are not pregnant or breastfeeding and for those wanting to lose weight.

The recipes in chapter 8 are tagged with the number of servings they supply from each food group to make it easier for you to meet the suggested daily amounts from each food group.

DAILY PORTIONS FROM EACH FOOD GROUP

Calorie Level: 1,600

Grains: 5 ounce-equivalents

Vegetables: 2 cups

Fruits: 1.5 cups

Dairy: 3 cups

Protein: 5 ounce-equivalents

Calorie Level: 1,800

Grains: 6 ounce-equivalents

Vegetables: 2.5 cups

Fruits: 1.5 cups

Dairy: 3 cups

Protein: 5 ounce-equivalents

Calorie Level: 2,000

Grains: 6 ounce-equivalents

Vegetables: 2.5 cups

Fruits: 2 cups

Dairy: 3 cups

Protein: 5.5 ounce-equivalents

Calorie Level: 2,200

Grains: 7 ounce-equivalents

Vegetables: 3 cups

Fruits: 2 cups

Dairy: 3 cups

Protein: 6 ounce-equivalents

Calorie Level: 2,400

Grains: 8 ounce-equivalents

Vegetables: 3 cups

Calorie Level: 2,400 (con't)

Fruits: 2 cups

Dairy: 3 cups

Protein: 6.5 ounce-equivalents

Calorie Level: 2,600

Grains: 9 ounce-equivalents

Vegetables: 3.5 cups

Fruits: 2 cups

Dairy: 3 cups

Protein: 6.5 ounce-equivalents

Calorie Level: 2,800

Grains: 10 ounce-equivalents

Vegetables: 3.5 cups

Fruits: 2.5 cups

Dairy: 3 cups

Protein: 7 ounce-equivalents

Calorie Level: 3,000

Grains: 10 ounce-equivalents

Vegetables: 4 cups

Fruits: 2.5 cups

Dairy: 3 cups

Protein: 7 ounce-equivalents

Calorie Level: 3,200

Grains: 10 ounce-equivalents

Vegetables: 4 cups

Fruits: 2.5 cups

Dairy: 3 cups

Protein: 7 ounce-equivalents

PREVENTING PORTION DISTORTION

When it comes to a balanced diet, portion size matters. Even when you're committed to eating healthfully, it's sometimes impossible to weigh and measure foods, and you may have little interest in doing so. That's OK. Portion control is literally at your fingertips when you consider that your hand is a convenient and portable method for estimating your portions.

- Your fist is equal to about 1 cup of cooked rice, pasta, other grains, veggies, or fruits.

- Your palm (flat) is about the size of 3 ounces of red meat, fish, or poultry, and 3 ounces of meat is about as thick as a deck of cards.

- Your palm (cupped) holds 1 ounce of nuts or raisins.

- A handful of chips, popcorn, or pretzels is about 2 ounces.

- Your thumb is about the size of 1 ounce of peanut butter or hard cheese.

- The tip of your thumb is about the size of one teaspoon of oil, mayonnaise, butter, or sugar.

THE FIVE FOOD GROUPS

Most foods, including chocolate bars, snack chips, and foot-long hot dogs, fit into a balanced diet, but such high-calorie, low-nutrient choices are not "everyday" foods. Eating nutrient-rich foods in the right portions is the key to controlling calories and getting the nutrients you need. This section delves into each of the five food groups in MyPlate. It explains why the foods are good for you and describes serving sizes so that you can get a good idea of what experts mean by a balanced eating plan.

THE GRAINS GROUP

Grains—such as those contained in bread, pasta, and rice—are a major source of carbohydrates, the body's preferred source of energy. Grains contain many nutrients, including the vitamins that help your body harness the energy from food and make it useful to you and your developing baby. Grains, particularly whole grains, also provide fiber, which promotes regular bowel movements and affords other benefits.

When you choose grains, pick whole-grain foods for at least half of the grain servings your MyPlate eating plan suggests, with a minimum of three a day. Whole grains—contained in whole-wheat bread, oatmeal, and brown rice, for example—are typically higher in fiber, certain vitamins and minerals, and phytonutrients than their refined counterparts (contained in white bread, many breakfast cereals, and white rice). Eating whole grains is linked to a lower risk of heart disease, cancer, and diabetes, and whole grains may be helpful with managing weight control before pregnancy as well as pregnancy weight gain because the fiber in whole grains helps to keep you fuller for longer.

A whole-grain product can be produced from any type of grain, including wheat, oats, corn, rice, and barley. Check the food label to be sure the food is made primarily from a whole grain. Ingredients are listed in descending order, so look for the word *whole* in front of the name of the grain as one of the first few ingredients. Take note: foods made only with bran may sound like whole-grain products, but they are not. Bran is just one part of a whole grain. When you are evaluating claims on food labels such as "made with whole grains," and the label gives the amount of whole grain in grams per serving, it's useful to know that the experts recommend at least 48 grams of whole grain daily.

REALITY CHECK: WHY SWEET TREATS AREN'T IN THE GRAINS GROUP

Cookies, cake, and other bakery foods are technically considered grains, but you won't find them on MyPlate's grain foods list because they are highly refined and contain too much added sugar and fat to be called nutrient-rich. Although grains with added fats and sugars can be part of a balanced eating plan, they should be "sometimes" foods. For example, a blueberry coffee-shop muffin can have four times as many calories as two slices of whole-wheat toast with blueberry jam, and far fewer nutrients.

The Food and Drug Administration regulates health claims made about food. A manufacturer may choose to include a health claim linking a food rich in whole grains to a reduced risk of heart disease and certain types of cancer, but that product must contain all portions of the grain kernel and a minimum of 51 percent whole grain by weight. The product must also meet specified levels for fat, cholesterol, and sodium.

While the emphasis is on choosing whole grains for half or more of your whole-grain intake, it's important to note that refined grains have some benefits. White bread, cereal, and pasta that are enriched provide added iron and four of the B vitamins, including folic acid.

In general, 1 slice of bread, 1 cup of ready-to-eat cereal, or $1/2$ cup of cooked rice, cooked pasta, or cooked cereal can be considered a 1 ounce-equivalent from the Grains Group. See the list below for grain foods and their portion sizes, which are equal to 1 ounce-equivalents.

Food	Amount Equal to 1 Ounce-Equivalent
Bagel	1 ounce (e.g., 1 mini)
Biscuits	1 small (2" in diameter)
Bread	1 regular slice or 1 small slice French or 4 snack-size slices
Cornbread	1 small piece ($2^1/2$" x $1^1/4$" x $1^1/4$")
Crackers	5 whole-wheat crackers or 2 rye crisp breads or 7 square or round crackers
English muffin	$1/2$ muffin
Grains, such as bulgur, quinoa, teff, barley, freekeh	$1/2$ cup cooked
Oatmeal (regular or quick-cooking)	$1/2$ cup cooked or 1 instant packet or 1 ounce ($1/3$ cup) dry
Pancakes	1 medium ($4^1/2$" in diameter) or 2 small (3" in diameter)
Pasta (includes couscous)	$1/2$ cup cooked or 1 ounce dry
Popcorn	3 cups popped

Ready-to-eat cereal	1 cup flakes or rounds or $1^1/_4$ cups puffed
Rice	$^1/_2$ cup cooked or 1 ounce dry
Tortillas	1 small (6") flour or corn

FROM THE RECIPE FILE

Quinoa is higher in protein than most grains, and it's versatile and convenient. Quinoa Salad with Toasted Pecans and Dried Apricots (page 292) is a tasty way to include more whole grains.

The Vegetable Group

Vegetables supply many nutrients, including fiber, potassium, vitamin C, and magnesium. Vegetables are not created equal, however. MyPlate divides vegetables into subgroups based on the nutrients they provide. For example, dark green leafy vegetables, including spinach, kale, and broccoli, offer the most vitamin K and provide vitamin C and folate; the red and orange vegetables have the most vitamin A (as carotenoids); and legumes (dried beans and peas) supply the highest fiber levels.

REALITY CHECK: IS VEGETABLE VARIETY CONFUSING YOU?

MyPlate recommends a variety of produce, which is illustrated by the five categories within the vegetable group. MyPlate even goes as far as suggesting how many servings to have from each subgroup over a seven-day period. By categorizing vegetables into subgroups and recommending how much to eat from each, MyPlate encourages variety, but also invites confusion. Here's the bottom line about vegetables: Pick vegetables that offer more fiber, vitamins, and minerals as well as less fat and fewer calories. For example, a medium baked potato supplies one and a half times the potassium of a medium order of fast-food french fries, with 223 fewer calories and 20 fewer grams of fat.

Dividing vegetables into groups doesn't mean that some are better for you than others, exactly. However, MyPlate recommends eating slightly more servings of vegetables such as carrots, tomatoes, and red bell pepper, over a week's time, compared to corn, green peas, and white potatoes, because red and orange vegetables tend to offer more nutrition for the calories. Corn, peas, potatoes, and winter squash are starchy vegetables, meaning they contain more carbohydrates and calories than the rest of the vegetables, which are considered nonstarchy. Nonstarchy vegetables are very low in calories and carbohydrates but rich in vitamins, minerals, and phytonutrients. Brightly colored vegetables are concentrated sources of vitamins, minerals, and fiber, but white and tan produce, including cauliflower, mushrooms, and onions, are chock-full of nutrition, too.

It may come as a surprise that dried beans and peas (such as garbanzo beans, soybeans, and black eyed peas) are listed in MyPlate's vegetable group as well as in the protein group. The reason is that dried beans and peas supply significant amounts of protein in addition to other nutrients.

In general, 1 cup of raw or cooked vegetables or vegetable juice or 2 cups of raw leafy greens can be considered 1 cup from the Vegetable Group. See the list below for how to count various types of vegetables based on a 1-cup serving:

Food	Amount Equal to 1 Cup
Dark Green Vegetables	
Broccoli	1 cup, chopped or florets OR 3 spears, 5" long, raw or cooked
Collard greens, mustard greens, turnip greens, and kale	1 cup, cooked
Raw leafy greens: spinach, romaine, watercress, dark green leafy lettuce, endive, escarole	2 cups, raw OR 1 cup, cooked
Red and Orange Vegetables	
Carrots	1 cup, raw or cooked, strips, slices, or chopped OR 2 medium, whole OR 1 cup, baby carrots (about 12)

Red and Orange Vegetables (cont.)

Pumpkin	1 cup, cooked and mashed
Red peppers	1 cup, chopped, raw, or cooked OR
	1 large pepper (3" diameter, $3^3/_4$" long)
Tomatoes	1 large raw whole (3") OR
	1 cup, chopped or sliced, raw, canned, or cooked
Tomato juice	1 cup
Sweet potato	1 large baked ($2^1/_4$" or more in diameter) OR
	1 cup, cooked, sliced or mashed
Winter squash (acorn, butternut, hubbard)	1 cup, cooked, cubed

Dry Beans and Peas

Dry beans and peas (such as black, garbanzo, kidney, pinto, soybeans, black-eyed, split, lentils)	1 cup, cooked, whole or mashed

Starchy Vegetables

Corn, yellow or white	1 cup
	1 large ear (8" to 9" long)
Green peas	1 cup
Potatoes	1 cup, diced or mashed OR
	1 medium, boiled or baked ($2^1/_2$" to 3" in diameter)
French fries	20 medium to long strips ($2^1/_2$" to 4" long)*

Other

Bean sprouts**	1 cup, cooked
Cabbage, green	1 cup, raw or cooked, chopped or shredded
Cauliflower	1 cup, pieces of florets, raw or cooked

Other (cont.)

Celery	1 cup, raw or cooked, diced or sliced, OR 2 large stalks (11" to 12" long)
Cucumbers	1 cup, raw, sliced or chopped
Green or wax beans	1 cup, cooked
Green peppers	1 cup, chopped, raw or cooked OR 1 large pepper (3" diameter, 3³/₄" long)
Lettuce, iceberg	2 cups, raw, shredded or chopped
Mushrooms	1 cup, raw or cooked
Onions	1 cup, raw or cooked
Summer squash or zucchini	1 cup, cooked, sliced or diced

*Contains added calories and should be consumed sparingly.

**Raw sprouts may contain harmful bacteria. Eat only cooked sprouts.

FROM THE RECIPE FILE

Make a double batch of Veggie "Stoup" (page 288).
Freeze half for later when you're too busy to prepare vegetables.

THE FRUIT GROUP

What's not to like about fruit? Fruit offers carbohydrates, fiber, potassium, vitamins A and C, and phytonutrients. Most fruit is bursting with fluid and supplies fiber, both of which are filling and may help with weight control. Fruit is naturally sweet and can help satisfy cravings for cookies, candy, and ice cream. Most fruit is easily portable and requires a minimum of preparation.

Fruits can be canned, frozen, whole, cut up, juiced, or pureed, but choose whole fruits most of the time. While 100 percent fruit juice can be part of a healthy eating plan, it has less fiber than whole fruits. Plus, it's easier to overdo it on juice, so you may get extra calories if you don't watch the portion size. Select fruits without added sugar, such as unsweetened applesauce or canned fruits packed in their natural juices rather than in syrup.

EAT FRUIT AT ANY TIME OF DAY

Fruit can be part of any meal or snack. Fruit's natural flavors pair well with vegetables in smoothies, in sandwiches (try sliced apple or pear in grilled cheese), and with meat or poultry, such as Chicken with Whole Wheat Couscous, Cranberries, and Almonds on page 248. Fruit is especially useful if you have a sweet tooth. Mango Ice "Milk" on page 303 supplies a cup of fruit with no added sugar!

In general, 1 cup of fruit or 100 percent fruit juice, or $^1/_2$ cup of dried fruit can be considered as 1 cup from the Fruit Group. Here are the fruit amounts that equal a 1-cup MyPlate serving.

Food	Amount Equal to 1 Cup
Apple	$^1/_2$ large (3$^1/_4$" in diameter) OR
	1 small (2$^1/_2$" in diameter) OR
	1 cup, raw or cooked, sliced or chopped
Applesauce	1 cup
Banana	1 large (8" to 9") OR 1 cup sliced
Berries (excluding strawberries)	1 cup
Cantaloupe	1 cup, diced or balls
Grapes	1 cup, whole or cut up OR 32 seedless grapes
Grapefruit	1 medium (4" in diameter) OR 1 cup sections
Mixed fruit (fruit cocktail)	1 cup, diced or sliced, raw or canned, drained
Orange	1 large (3" in diameter) OR 1 cup sections
Orange, mandarin	1 cup, canned, drained
Peach	1 large (2$^3/_4$" in diameter) OR
	1 cup, raw, cooked, or canned and drained, sliced or diced OR
	2 halves, canned
Pear	1 medium pear (2$^1/_2$ per pound) OR
	1 cup, raw, cooked, or canned and drained, sliced or diced

Pineapple	1 cup, raw, cooked, or canned and drained, chunks, sliced, or crushed
Plum	1 cup, sliced, raw or cooked OR
	3 medium OR
	2 large plums
Strawberries	About 8 large berries OR
	1 cup, fresh or frozen, whole, halved, or sliced
Watermelon	1 small wedge (1" thick) or 1 cup, diced or balls
Dried fruit	$1/2$ cup
100% fruit juice (orange, apple, grape, grapefruit, etc.)	1 cup

THE DAIRY GROUP

The members of the milk group provide many nutrients, including protein, phosphorus, and potassium. Milk products are probably best known for containing calcium and vitamin D, but fortified milk is the only reliable dairy source of both. Vitamin D is added to cow's milk and many plant milks, and also to some brands of yogurt. Cheese typically lacks vitamin D. Soy beverages fortified with calcium, vitamin A, and vitamin D are included as part of the dairy group because they are similar to cow's milk based on their nutrient composition.

MyPlate's dairy recommendations for adults are the easiest of all to remember: 3 cups of milk daily or the equivalent in dairy foods, no matter what calorie level you've chosen for yourself, whether you're pregnant or not, or breastfeeding (and it's the same for men, too). Milk-based desserts are included in MyPlate's dairy group, but they contain added sugar, fat, or both, so you would need to eat more of them to get the same nutrients as other lower-calorie options in the group. (Sour cream and cream cheese aren't in the dairy group because they don't contain enough calcium to qualify.) Reach for fat-free and low-fat dairy foods most of the time to limit saturated fat intake and to get more nutrients for the calories. For example, you *could* choose three servings of ice cream every day to satisfy your dairy food requirements, but it would "cost" you far more in calories, added sugar, and saturated fat than choosing low-fat or fat-free milk and yogurt and reduced-fat cheese.

WHICH MILK IS RIGHT FOR YOU?

"Drink your milk" has been a favorite refrain of parents for decades. Until the recent past, mom and dad were probably referring to cow's milk. While cow's milk is still the most popular type, plant "milks," including almond, rice, coconut, hemp, and cashew, are gaining ground. Plant milks are a boon for people who cannot tolerate cow's milk, as are lactose-free and lactose-reduced cow's milks. People who choose not to drink cow's milk may turn to plant milks, but it's important to note that plant milks don't offer the same nutrition, and they are not included in the MyPlate dairy group. Fortified soy milk is the exception. Protein levels vary in plant milks. For example, 8 ounces of rice milk has 1 gram of protein while the same amount of cow's milk has 8 grams. Many plant milk products are fortified with calcium and other nutrients, but they may not be absorbed as well by the body as what's found naturally in cow's milk. Sweetened versions of plant milks also contain added sugars.

In general, 1 cup of milk, yogurt, or soy milk (soy beverage), $1^{1}/_{2}$ ounces of natural cheese, or 2 ounces of processed cheese can be considered as 1 cup from the Dairy Group. See the list below for servings in the milk group.

Food	Amount Equal to 1 Cup
Milk	1 cup OR $^{1}/_{2}$-pint container (including lactose-free) OR
	$^{1}/_{2}$ cup evaporated milk
Yogurt*	1 cup (8 ounces)
Cheese	$1^{1}/_{2}$ ounces hard cheese, such as cheddar, mozzarella, Swiss, or Parmesan

	$1/3$ cup shredded cheese
	2 ounces processed cheese (e.g., American)
	$1/2$ cup ricotta cheese
	2 cups cottage cheese
Milk-based desserts	1 cup pudding made with milk
	1 cup frozen yogurt
	$1^1/2$ cups ice cream
Soy milk	1 cup OR $1/2$-pint container calcium-fortified soy milk

*Single-serve yogurt containers are often 6 ounces or less, which count as just $3/4$ cup of dairy.

FROM THE RECIPE FILE

Artichoke Quiche with Thyme and Gruyere Cheese (page 254) is an entrée that serves up substantial calcium as well as protein and some fiber.

PROTEIN FOODS

Meat, poultry, fish, beans and peas (legumes), eggs, soy products, nuts, seeds, and products made from them, are all part of MyPlate's protein foods group. The members of the protein group are diverse, and they offer an array of nutrients. Protein is what brings them together, and the idea is to select a variety of protein foods, including at least 8 ounces of fish (two meals) each week if you're not pregnant and 8 to 12 ounces of fish (two to three meals) a week when pregnant or breastfeeding. See chapter 6 for more about choosing fish and seafood.

FROM THE RECIPE FILE

You don't have to go meatless to include more plant foods. Chicken and White Bean Chili (page 286) is a good example of how to mix and match poultry and beans to include the protein you need.

Every protein group member has a lot to offer, nutrition-wise. For example, among other nutrients, fish and shellfish are rich in brain-building and heart-healthy omega-3 fats; meat and poultry supply iron and B vitamins; and beans and peas are rich in fiber and folate. The majority of your protein servings should be foods that are relatively low in saturated fat, such as lean ground beef, skinless poultry, seafood, and legumes.

ABOUT BEANS AND PEAS

Beans and peas are legumes. Legumes include kidney beans, pinto beans, black beans, lima beans, black-eyed peas, garbanzo beans (chickpeas), split peas, and lentils. You may think beans and peas are for vegetarians only, but they're for all types of eaters! Even better, legumes are part of MyPlate's vegetable group as well as the protein group. That means they do double duty in a balanced eating plan.

In general, 1 ounce of meat, poultry, or fish, $1/4$ cup cooked beans, one egg, 1 tablespoon of peanut butter, or $1/2$ ounce of nuts or seeds can be considered as 1 ounce-equivalent from the Protein Foods Group. Here are the offerings from the protein group:

Food	Amount Equal to 1 Ounce
Lean cooked beef, cooked ham, or pork	1 ounce
Cooked chicken or turkey, without skin	1 ounce
Sliced turkey sandwich meat	1 ounce
Cooked fish or shellfish	1 ounce
Eggs*	1 whole
Nuts	$1/2$ ounce (12 almonds, 24 pistachios, or 7 walnut halves)
Seeds (pumpkin, sunflower, or squash)	$1/2$ ounce
Almond butter	1 tablespoon

Peanut butter	1 tablespoon
Beans and peas (black beans, kidney beans, white beans, etc., or chickpeas, lentils, or split peas, etc.)	$1/4$ cup cooked
Baked beans, refried beans	$1/4$ cup
Tofu	$1/4$ cup (about 2 ounces)
Tempeh	1 ounce cooked
Roasted soybeans	$1/4$ cup
Falafel patty	1 ($2^1/4$" or about 4 ounces)
Hummus	2 tablespoons

*3 egg whites equal 2 ounce-equivalents of protein. Note that all the vitamins and minerals, and nearly half the protein, is found in egg yolks.

MAKE ROOM FOR FAVORITE FOODS

You're eating five servings of fruits and vegetables every day, and you're also achieving the suggested intakes for low-fat dairy foods, lean protein sources, and whole grains. Is there any room for fries, chips, and sweets in MyPlate's plan for healthy eating? You bet! No matter how many calories you're eating to lose weight, maintain it, or gain it, there's some room for extras—anywhere from 130 calories to upwards of 600 calories, depending on your daily calorie needs, which could be higher than other plans because of physical activity and other factors. These extra calories are left over after you have satisfied your nutrient needs by choosing the suggested amounts of nutrient-rich foods from each of the food groups. You can spend leftover calories on any food you like—as long as it's safe, that is, especially during pregnancy and breastfeeding. For example, a 2,000-calorie USDA Healthy-Eating Pattern allows for nearly 300 calories to spend any way you like. You can use them on extra bread or meat, or on three crème-filled sandwich cookies and 8 ounces of 1% low-fat milk, but it's always wiser to stick with healthier choices.

FATS AND OILS

The fat in food makes it taste good and makes eating more satisfying. Although technically not a food group, oils, such as canola, olive, and safflower oils, are part of a healthy eating pattern. Oils are the major source of essential fatty acids that your body cannot make, and they supply vitamin E. Oils are also naturally present in nuts, seeds, seafood, olives, and avocados.

Most oils are rich in unsaturated fats, or the healthy fats. The fat in some tropical oils, such as coconut, palm kernel oil, and palm oil, are not included in the oils group because they are high in saturated fat, which is bad for your heart.

Most of the time, oils, such as canola and olive, should be used in place of solid fats, such as butter and lard. Oils come from many different plants, and from seafood. A number of foods are naturally high in oils, like nuts, olives, fish, and avocados. Foods that are mainly composed of oil include mayonnaise, certain salad dressings, and soft margarine with no trans fat.

The suggested amount for oils on a 2,000-calorie eating plan is about 5 teaspoons per day, or 27 grams. Some of us get enough oil in the foods we eat, including nuts, fish, cooking oils, and salad dressings.

SAMPLE MEAL PLANS

Now you know what to eat, but perhaps you're perplexed about how it all fits together. These suggested sample meal plans, which use recommendations from MyPlate, provide you with ideas of how to put together a balanced eating plan.

1,600 Calories (For Weight Loss in Sedentary Individuals Who Are Not Pregnant or Breastfeeding)

Breakfast
1 cup ready-to-eat whole-grain cereal or $1/2$ cup cooked oatmeal
1 cup fat-free or 1% low-fat milk
$1/2$ medium banana
1 hard-cooked egg

Lunch
Salad: 2 ounces cooked boneless, skinless chicken or turkey; 1 cup dark green leafy vegetables, such as romaine lettuce or baby spinach; 2 tablespoons canned, drained beans, such as black beans; $1/2$ cup chopped tomato. Top with 1 teaspoon olive oil and balsamic vinegar.
1-ounce whole-grain roll
1 cup fat-free or 1% low-fat milk

Snack
$1^1/2$ ounces hard cheese, such as cheddar
1 mini (1 ounce) whole-grain bagel

Dinner
3 ounces cooked salmon, pork tenderloin, or lean beef
1 cup cooked brown rice or quinoa with 1 teaspoon trans fat–free tub margarine or olive oil
1 cup cooked broccoli with 1 teaspoon trans fat–free tub margarine or olive oil

Snack
1 cup plain low-fat yogurt mixed with 1 medium chopped apple or pear, pinch of ground cinnamon, and sweetener of your choice

2,000 Calories (For Adults Who Are Moderately Active and Not Pregnant or Breastfeeding)

Breakfast
1 cup ready-to-eat whole-grain cereal or $^1/_2$ cup cooked oatmeal
1 cup fat-free or 1% low-fat milk
1 medium banana
1 hard-cooked egg

Lunch
Salad: 2 ounces cooked boneless, skinless chicken or turkey; 2 cups
    dark leafy green vegetables; 2 tablespoons canned, drained beans,
    such as black beans; $^1/_2$ cup chopped tomato. Top with 2 teaspoons
    olive oil and balsamic vinegar.
1-ounce whole-grain roll
1 cup plain low-fat yogurt mixed with 1 medium chopped apple
    or pear, pinch of ground cinnamon, and sweetener of your choice

Snack
$1^1/_2$ ounces hard cheese, such as cheddar
7 soda crackers
12 baby carrots

Dinner
3 ounces cooked salmon, pork tenderloin, or lean beef
1 cup cooked brown rice or quinoa with 1 teaspoon trans fat–free
    tub margarine
1 cup cooked broccoli with 1 teaspoon trans fat–free tub margarine
    or olive oil

Snack
3 cups low-fat popcorn, popped

2,400 Calories (For Many Pregnant or Breastfeeding Women Who Are Moderately Active)

Breakfast

1 cup ready-to-eat whole-grain cereal or $1/2$ cup cooked oatmeal

1 cup fat-free or 1% low-fat milk

1 slice whole-grain toast with 1 teaspoon peanut butter or almond butter

1 medium banana

1 hard-cooked egg

Lunch

Salad: 2 ounces cooked boneless, skinless chicken or turkey; 2 cups dark leafy green vegetables; $1/2$ cup canned, drained beans, such as black beans; $1/2$ cup chopped tomato. Top with 2 teaspoons olive oil and balsamic vinegar.

2-ounce whole-grain roll

1 cup plain low-fat yogurt mixed with 1 medium chopped apple or pear, pinch of ground cinnamon, and sweetener of your choice

Snack

$1 1/2$ ounces hard cheese, such as cheddar

7 soda crackers

12 baby carrots

Dinner

4 ounces cooked salmon, pork tenderloin, or lean beef

1 cup cooked brown rice or quinoa with 1 teaspoon trans fat–free tub margarine

1 cup cooked broccoli with 1 teaspoon trans fat–free tub margarine or olive oil

Snack

3 cups low-fat popcorn, popped

REALITY CHECK: POLICE YOUR PORTIONS

Do you really have to weigh and measure all your food to eat a healthy diet? No, but it helps, especially when you don't have a clue about suggested serving sizes and also when you suspect that you're overdoing it on portions. Refer to the picture of MyPlate on page 90 to get a visual reminder of what to put on your plate.

WHEN SHOULD YOU EAT?

Is it better to eat six times a day or three? Will you gain weight if you consume most of your calories in the evening? What's the best way to eat to maximize energy? These are common questions and valid concerns, especially when you're pregnant or thinking about having a baby, breastfeeding, or trying to shed pounds.

It's best to spread out meals and snacks during the day to provide your body with the energy it needs; eating three, four, or even six meals is fine, as long as you eat the right amount of food for you. Many people skimp on eating during the day and save most of their food for dinner and afterward. You won't automatically gain weight by leaving the bulk of your eating until evening, but you might overdo it. After a long day, it's often too tiring to police yourself, and it's easier to lose control of portions.

Women in their second and third trimesters of pregnancy and those who are breastfeeding may feel the need to eat more often throughout the day because their energy demands are higher. As pregnancy progresses, it will probably feel better to divide your food intake into smaller, more frequent meals.

13 SUPER FOODS THAT MAKE GOOD HEALTH TASTE GREAT

MyPlate encourages nutrient-rich choices because they provide the most nutrients for the calories. The following foods are among some of the most nutrient-rich picks for moms and expectant mothers. You'll find recipes for these and other fantastic foods in chapter 8.

AVOCADO: Avocados supply heart-healthy fat, fiber, and folate in addition to several other vitamins and minerals. They are also rich in phytonutrients, plant compounds that support good health.

How to use: Cut in half, and eat with a spoon! Add to salads, and used smashed avocado instead of mayonnaise in sandwiches. Add to smoothies and desserts.

BEEF: Lean beef is rich in protein; the B vitamins niacin (vitamin B3), B6, and B12; and zinc and iron in highly absorbable forms. Beef is also an excellent source of choline, which is required for proper brain development and for possibly preventing neural tube defects.

How to use: Add cooked, crumbled 95 percent lean ground beef to pasta sauce; use it in tacos, for burgers, in stir-fry dishes, and in chili. Use lean cuts of beef for soups and stews.

BERRIES: Don't be fooled by their small size. Berries are nutritional powerhouses. Berries are rich in potassium, folate, fiber, fluid, carbohydrates, and vitamin C. The phytonutrients in berries protect cells from damage.

How to use: Top whole-grain cereal with berries; use berries in smoothies made with yogurt or milk, in pancakes and other quick breads, and in salads; eat plain as a snack.

BROCCOLI: Broccoli provides folate, fiber, and calcium; lutein, zeaxanthin, and carotenoids (which bolster vision); and potassium (for fluid balance and normal blood pressure). Broccoli also contains the raw materials for vitamin A production in your body and your baby's body.

How to use: Add broccoli to pasta and stir-fry dishes; enjoy it steamed and topped with a smattering of olive oil; puree cooked broccoli and add to soups. Lightly coat bite-size pieces with olive oil and roast for about fifteen minutes on a baking sheet at 400°F until tender.

CHEESE: Cheese supplies concentrated amounts of calcium (for your bones and your baby's bones) as well as vitamin B12 and protein. Reduced-fat varieties, such as cheddar and part-skim mozzarella, save on calories, fat, and cholesterol.

How to use: Eat cheese as a snack with whole-grain crackers or fruit; sprinkle grated cheese on top of soups; and add cheese to salads, sandwiches, and omelets.

EGGS: Eggs provide all the amino acids that you and your baby need to thrive. Eggs supply more than a dozen vitamins and minerals as well as other nutrients, including choline (for brain development and preventing birth defects) and lutein and zeaxanthin (for healthy eyesight). Certain brands of eggs supply the omega-3 fats that your baby needs for proper brain development and peak vision; check the label to be sure you're getting docosahexaenoic acid (DHA) for the most benefit.

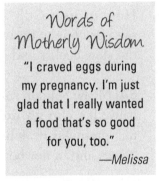

Words of Motherly Wisdom

"I craved eggs during my pregnancy. I'm just glad that I really wanted a food that's so good for you, too."

—Melissa

How to use: Enjoy eggs in omelets and frittatas; hard-cooked in salads and sandwiches or as a snack; and as part of homemade waffles, crepes, and whole-grain French toast.

LEGUMES: Chickpeas, lentils, black beans, soybeans, and other beans supply fiber, protein, iron, folate, calcium, and zinc.

How to use: Include them in chili, soups, salads, and pasta dishes; as hummus with whole-grain crackers; and as a filling in wrap sandwiches.

MILK: Milk is an excellent source of calcium, phosphorus, and vitamin D—bone-building nutrients that a mother and her child require every day. Milk is also rich in protein, vitamin A, and several B vitamins.

How to use: Drink plain or flavored milk; use milk to make hot chocolate; include it in smoothies made with fruit; top whole-grain cereal and fruit with it; and use it in pudding. Prepare oatmeal in the microwave with milk instead of water to include a serving of dairy foods.

PORK TENDERLOIN: Are you tired of chicken? Pork tenderloin is even leaner than skinless chicken breast. Pork supplies several B vitamins as well as protein, iron, zinc, and choline.

How to use: Grill, broil, or bake pork tenderloin. Serve with salsa or chunky unsweetened applesauce. Make pulled pork in the slow cooker and serve on whole-grain buns.

SALMON: Salmon supplies high-quality protein to you and your baby. It's also an excellent source of DHA, the omega-3 fat that promotes peak brain development and vision in developing babies and in newborns.

How to use: Grill or broil salmon, and use canned or pouched salmon in salads, sandwiches, burgers, and pasta dishes.

SWEET POTATO: Sweet potatoes provide vitamin C, folate, fiber, and carotenoids (compounds that your body converts to vitamin A). Sweet potatoes also supply potassium in large amounts.

How to use: Sweet potatoes are delicious when baked. They can be eaten cold as snacks or warm as side dishes. Mash cooked, peeled sweet potatoes with orange juice. You can also roast them as follows: slice peeled sweet potatoes into wedges, coat lightly with canola oil and salt, and roast on a baking sheet at 400°F until tender, about fifteen to twenty minutes.

WHOLE GRAINS: Whole grains contain more fiber and trace nutrients than the processed grains you'll find in foods like white bread, white rice, and white flour. Enriched whole grains are fortified with folic acid and other B vitamins, iron, and zinc.

How to use: Have oatmeal for breakfast; use whole-grain breads for sandwiches; make brown rice, wild rice, whole-wheat pasta (including whole-wheat couscous), farro, quinoa or freekeh as a side dish or salad; and snack on popcorn or whole-grain crackers.

YOGURT (plain, low-fat, or fat-free): Yogurt supplies protein, calcium, B vitamins, and zinc; some brands also supply vitamin D, so check the label. Greek yogurt has more protein but less calcium than regular yogurt. Plain yogurt of any type contains more calcium than milk and flavored yogurt.

How to use: Combine plain yogurt with fruit preserves or honey, fresh or dried fruit, or crunchy whole-grain cereal. Use plain or vanilla yogurt to top cooked sweet potatoes or for smoothies.

MOVING ON

You can see by the way MyPlate is organized that all of the food groups work together to provide a balanced nutrient intake. Hopefully, you have a better understanding of an eating plan that best suits you, whether you are waiting for pregnancy, are pregnant, or are breastfeeding. There's no need to expect to eat "perfectly," even when you use MyPlate as a plan for a balanced diet. Try to come as close as possible to the suggested daily amounts, and include a variety of delicious foods every day.

We're moving on! The next chapter delves into the details of nutrition during pregnancy and all its stages. You'll learn about what your body is going through, or will go through, how your baby grows, and what to expect on the nine-month journey to delivery.

4

Your Pregnancy: Expect the Best

Hooray! You're having a baby! Maybe you've waited for this to happen for a long time—or perhaps you weren't anticipating pregnancy so soon. Whatever the case, healthy habits and regular visits to a licensed health care professional, such as an obstetrician or a certified nurse-midwife, will help you have the healthiest child possible.

You'll want to know what's going on every step of the way from now until delivery day. This chapter delves into how nutrition and physical activity influence your child's development—and your well-being—during each trimester.

THE FIRST TRIMESTER (WEEKS ONE TO THIRTEEN)

Your pregnancy may not yet be obvious to others, but you may be feeling the effects. An abundance of pregnancy hormones that support implantation, the growth of the uterus and the placenta, and the expansion of your circulatory system during early pregnancy can be constant reminders that you're expecting.

At the beginning of pregnancy, you may experience tender breasts, frequent urination, rapid changes in blood pressure, extreme emotions, bouts of unexpected fatigue, intense hunger, a heightened sensitivity to smells, and so-called morning sickness that can last all day. These effects of pregnancy differ among women, and they occur at different times after conceiving, sometimes sooner rather than later. You probably won't experience all these pregnancy changes, and even when you do they could be mild.

So, what's going on with baby? A lot!

After sperm and egg meet up, about six days pass before the embryo implants into the lining of the uterus, or womb. Once an embryo has secured itself in the womb, it starts receiving a supply of blood, which contains oxygen and nutrients, from your body. The cells of the embryo, which are multiplying very quickly, begin to differentiate (that is, develop specific functions) soon after implantation. The process of differentiation produces specialized cells that organize themselves into tissues and organs, such as the brain, the heart, the liver, and the circulatory system.

Tissues and organs develop on a tight timetable during the first trimester, but they don't all take shape at the same rate during these initial thirteen weeks. By the time the second trimester starts, all cell differentiation is complete, which is why experts say the first trimester lays the foundation for your child's well-being later on. When you know you're expecting, you can do your best to include the foods and nutrients you need and avoid substances considered harmful during pregnancy.

What to Eat Now

You're eating for two, but not for two adults, so there's no need to double your calorie intake! This may sound surprising, but you don't need any extra calories during the first trimester. The baby is small—weighing only about an ounce by the end of twelve weeks—and fetal growth, though quite rapid, does not require additional energy. However, the daily quotas for several important nutrients, including folic acid, increase. That's why, as always, it's important to make the most nutrient-rich food choices you can. Stick with your MyPlate Prepregnancy Eating Plan until the second trimester starts. See chapter 3 for how to get started on a healthy eating plan.

Although you don't actually need additional calories, if you feel hungrier than usual during the first trimester, there's no reason to deprive yourself, as long as you select healthy foods most of the time. Avoid using your pregnancy as a reason to overeat or to indulge in large portions of higher-calorie foods with few nutrients, including cookies, french fries, and snack chips.

You may gain between one and about five pounds during the first trimester, and you might not gain any weight if you're queasy with so-called "morning sickness" that lasts most of the day. Your health care provider will weigh you at your first prenatal visit and at every visit until delivery day. Recording your weight on a regular basis helps your health care team determine whether you're putting on the right number of pounds for you to promote a healthy birth weight in your baby. It also alerts them to big decreases or increases in weight that could signal health problems. Unless you're told otherwise, there's probably no need to weigh yourself at home between visits, because your weight can fluctuate, and small changes on the scale have little to do with overall pregnancy weight gain. If you were trying to drop some pounds before pregnancy, put off that goal until after the baby is born. Pregnancy is no time to try to lose weight.

REALITY CHECK: WHEN WEIGHT GAIN IS WORRISOME

Some women who have struggled with disordered eating in the past, or who are struggling with it when they conceive, may be fearful of pregnancy weight gain. It's important to discuss your feelings about your weight with a qualified health care expert. It might be worthwhile to speak with a mental health professional and a registered dietitian nutritionist (RDN) who specializes in disordered eating.

If you're pregnant with twins or triplets, don't wait until the second trimester to increase food intake. Plan on adding more calories as soon as you find out you're having more than one baby. (See chapter 3 for more about calorie needs for twin pregnancies.) The intention is to maximize your baby's birth weight. Women pregnant with more than one baby tend to deliver earlier, and eating more food starting in the first trimester increases the chances that your babies' weight at birth will be closer to normal, even if they are preterm.

Take Care of Yourself

If you haven't already done so, stop smoking cigarettes, and quit alcohol and recreational drugs, including the illegal, legal, and prescription kinds. Using these substances during pregnancy increases the risk for low-birth-weight and preterm infants, and for many other problems.

Steer clear of all acne and skin treatments that contain vitamin A. (See page 21 for more about vitamin A-containing medications.) However, do not suddenly stop taking medications that treat chronic conditions, including depression, asthma, diabetes, and thyroid disease. Tell the health care providers who help you to manage these conditions about your pregnancy so you can proceed in the safest manner. While you're at it, check every medication you take with your doctor or pharmacist for its safety during pregnancy,

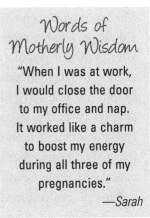

Words of
Motherly Wisdom

"When I was at work, I would close the door to my office and nap. It worked like a charm to boost my energy during all three of my pregnancies."
—*Sarah*

including common over-the-counter painkillers, cold medicines, and anti-inflammatory drugs, such as ibuprofen.

EATING LESS, GAINING WEIGHT

You're nauseated nearly all day long. You can't stand the sight or smell of most of your favorite foods. It's tough to even remember when you last ate a balanced meal. Nevertheless, you're gaining weight. What gives? It's possible to put on pounds during the first trimester even when your appetite is nonexistent. Pregnancy hormones promote fluid retention, which can cause some weight gain. You might also be less active than normal, which could be responsible for a few pregnancy pounds, too.

Try as much as possible to pamper yourself, especially if you are fatigued or experience nausea or vomiting or both. (See chapter 7 for more on "morning sickness.") Avoid unnecessary stress like additional responsibilities at work or an overwhelming home-renovation project.

Ask for help, and allow your spouse or partner and others to shoulder some of the responsibility of cooking and cleaning. Get plenty of rest when you can, even if it means putting your head down on your desk at work to take a catnap during your lunch hour!

Do You Need a Prenatal Supplement?

Most women receive a prescription from their health care provider for a daily prenatal vitamin, which also includes key minerals, immediately after getting a positive pregnancy test. Prescribing prenatal vitamins is such a widespread practice that you might be surprised to learn that experts do not agree that all women need a prescription or over-the-counter (OTC) prenatal pill. However, there are many reasons to take prenatal vitamins before, during, and after pregnancy, including the fact that nobody eats a perfect diet every day and that even a balanced pregnancy eating plan can fall short for certain nutrients, particularly iron.

Vitamin and mineral pills, often called "multis," are not substitutes for a healthy diet at any time of life. However, they are capable of filling gaps for nutrients, such as folic acid and iron, that promote good health for you and your growing child. You may choose to take a prescription or OTC prenatal supplement, or a regular multivitamin. Of course, you can also opt out of taking any supplements. It's up to you.

You're a good candidate for prescription prenatals, which will often contain more nutrients than an OTC supplement, if your diet was poor at the outset of your pregnancy or has been at any time during the pregnancy, or if your diet had been inadequate for months prior to conception. Women who are carrying more than one baby will benefit from a prescription prenatal supplement, and so will those with certain chronic conditions. Women who have had a pregnancy affected by a neural tube defect such as spina bifida should speak with their doctor before conception for prescription-level doses of folic acid to take before conceiving and during pregnancy.

> ### Words of Motherly Wisdom
> "I could not take the large prenatal pills, so I took children's chewables instead."
> —Janice

Even when you include a variety of foods and your eating pattern is balanced, it's a good idea to take at least an OTC daily multi with about 100 percent of the Daily Value (DV) for iron and folic acid prior to and during pregnancy, throughout breastfeeding, and afterward. If you decide on an OTC supplement, choose one with mostly beta-carotene as its source of vitamin A, and one that does not exceed 3,000 micrograms (mcg) or 10,000 International Units (IU) of vitamin A. Since you'll likely be eating foods with vitamin A and beta-carotene, it's perfectly fine to choose a supplement with even less vitamin A. Make sure your multi supplies 600 mcg of folic acid, which is the recommended amount for pregnancy, at least 27 milligrams of iron, and 150 mcg iodine. (See "All About Iron," below.) Also, to avoid overdoing it on vitamins and minerals, don't take an OTC multivitamin and a prescription prenatal pill simultaneously.

All About Iron

Iron requirements increase significantly during pregnancy. Your body ramps up its red blood cell production to support your growing baby, and red blood cells require iron. The body gets the iron it needs from your diet and the iron stored in your body, which you must replenish so that you don't become depleted. It's next to impossible for most women to reach the suggested intake of 27 milligrams (mg) of iron during pregnancy with food alone. The Centers for Disease Control and Prevention recommends that all pregnant women take 30 mg of iron either as an individual supplement or as part of a prenatal vitamin, which is slightly higher than the 27 mg per day Dietary Reference Intake for iron determined by the Institute of Medicine. Prescription and OTC prenatal vitamins often contain adequate iron for pregnancy, but check to see if yours has at least 27 mg. After testing your blood to determine iron stores, your doctor may recommend an additional 60 to 120 mg of iron a day to correct insufficient iron levels in your body.

Although some experts contend that it's not necessary to take the large doses of iron found in prescription and OTC prenatal supplements if you are not iron-deficient, many women have low iron stores well before conception, so taking extra iron during pregnancy typically makes sense. There is rarely a need to take prescription-strength prenatal vitamins

before conceiving or after delivery, although many physicians may prescribe them.

THE PROBLEM WITH PRENATAL VITAMINS

It's possible that you won't be able to tolerate the pills your doctor has
prescribed, because they are large and difficult to swallow for some
women, or because the high levels of iron can cause an upset stomach,
diarrhea, or constipation, or all of the above! Tell your health care provider if you are having problems taking a prenatal vitamin. You might be
able to switch to a smaller pill with less iron, pills with a slicker coating
to make them go down more easily, or a regular, liquid, or chewable
vitamin with iron. If constipation is troubling you, follow a high-fiber
eating plan and drink plenty of fluids. Take your supplement at night or
after meals to avoid queasiness, or cut it in half to split up the dosage
during the day.

Choosing Prenatal Dietary Supplements

You may choose to forgo prescription prenatal supplements for the OTC
variety. There are no official recommendations for what should be in
prenatal supplements, so they often vary by manufacturer. The following table is meant to guide your choice of a supplement for pregnancy
and breastfeeding. It's particularly important for vegans to get enough
iron and vitamin B12 from dietary supplements, supplemented foods,
or a combination. Teens may need more of some of the nutrients listed
below. See the discussions of the individual nutrients in chapter 3 for a
teenager's specific needs.

DAILY VITAMIN AND MINERAL NEEDS

Nutrient	Pregnancy (19–50 years old)	Breastfeeding (19–50 years old)
Vitamin A*, mcg	770 (2,541 IU)	1,300 (4,290 IU)
Vitamin C, mg	85	120

Vitamin D, IU	600	600
Vitamin E, IU	22 (15 mg)	28 (19 mg)
Vitamin K, mcg	90	90
Vitamin B1 (thiamin), mg	1.4	1.4
Vitamin B2 (riboflavin), mg	1.4	1.6
Vitamin B3 (niacin), mg	18	17
Vitamin B5 (pantothenic acid)	6	7
Vitamin B6, mg	1.9	2
Folate, mcg	600	500
Vitamin B12, mcg	2.6	2.8
Calcium**, mg	1,000	1,000
Iodine, mcg	220	290
Iron, mg	27	9
Magnesium, mg	350	310
Zinc, mg	11	12

Mcg = micrograms, mg = milligrams, and IU = International Units

*Choose a supplement with most of the vitamin A as beta-carotene. Do not exceed 3,000 mcg (10,000 IU) of vitamin A on a daily basis during pregnancy.

**Multivitamin/mineral supplements are generally low in calcium, so you may need an additional calcium supplement if you don't get enough calcium from foods.

DHA Supplements

Many prenatal vitamins don't include DHA, the omega-3 fat that is important for the development of your baby's brain, nerves, and eyes. The recommended intake for DHA during pregnancy and breastfeeding is at least 200 mg a day. Eating the suggested two to three fish meals a week (8 to 12 ounces) will help you meet your DHA needs. If you don't get enough DHA from fish and other fortified foods (see page 50), consider taking a daily DHA supplement.

You Can Have Too Much of a Good Thing

Many foods are fortified with vitamins and minerals. Depending on your selections, it's easy to consume more than the suggested amounts for certain nutrients, especially if you are also taking an OTC or a prescription prenatal supplement, which supplies at least 100 percent, and often far more, of your daily vitamin and mineral needs.

Foods designed for pregnant and nursing women are often touted as providing all the necessary nutrients for pregnancy and for breastfeeding, but their nutrition profile can be more like a multivitamin supplement than food. Snack bars and nutrition drinks tend to contain added B vitamins, particularly folic acid. For example, your favorite pregnancy snack bar may contain 800 mcg of folic acid. Add this to the folic acid in your prescription prenatal pill (typically 1,000 mcg) and in the bowl of fortified cereal (400 mcg) you eat for breakfast, and you'd be taking in at least 2,200 mcg of folic acid a day when you need only about one-fourth that amount. Excess folic acid could cause a type of anemia. Check the Nutrition Facts panel of the processed foods you eat on a regular basis to see if you are overdoing it for vitamins and minerals. Limit highly fortified convenience foods, and focus on including whole foods and a daily multivitamin and mineral supplement.

Outsmarting a Poor Appetite: Stealth Nutrition

Just a few weeks ago, in your prepregnancy life, you might have adored Chinese food, couldn't begin the day without a giant cup of steaming hot coffee, and wouldn't think of passing up dark chocolate. Now you're repulsed at the thought of your favorite foods.

Food aversions—and their counterparts, food cravings (see the section on the second trimester in this chapter)—are most likely the result of pregnancy hormones. The hormonal surges that are brought on by pregnancy intensify your sense of smell, which heavily influences food preferences.

The only certainty about food aversions is their changeability. Food preferences tend to differ from pregnancy to pregnancy. That's why you might have loved sirloin steak during your first pregnancy, but you can't bear the sight (or smell!) of it now. Even more puzzling is that food preferences can change on a daily basis. Pregnancy has even been known to alter a woman's preference for certain foods for years, and sometimes, indefinitely.

Avoiding certain foods or entire food groups can become problematic, especially if you continue to shy away from them well into the second and third trimesters and you aren't making up for the nutrients (including calories, fat, and protein) that you're missing. The negative effects of food aversions on nutrient intake are intensified when you're unable to take a daily vitamin and mineral supplement because of morning sickness.

Here are some tips for sneaking in the nutrition you may be missing:

- Include mild-tasting vegetables, such as mashed white or sweet potatoes and green beans. Puree cooked legumes, such as canned garbanzo beans, and stronger-smelling vegetables, such as broccoli and cauliflower, and use in soups and as side dishes or sauces for meat.

- Have cold entrees, like sandwiches, instead of hot dishes. Warm foods are more aromatic and can cause nausea.

- Try all-fruit or fruit-and-vegetable smoothies (pureed sweet potato, beets, and canned pumpkin pair well with fruit) when you can't stand the thought of drinking plain milk or soy beverages, eating fruit or vegetables, or all of the above.

- If meat is making you gag, turn to beans, soy foods such as tofu, nuts, nut butters, reduced-fat cheese or Greek yogurt for protein and other nutrients. Stir textured vegetable protein crumbles (made from soy) or pureed cottage cheese into warm pasta sauce, or add pureed cooked beans to soups and stews. Consider adding whey protein powder, dry milk powder, or peanut powder to smoothies and warm dishes, such as oatmeal, for more protein.

> ***Words of Motherly Wisdom***
>
> "When I was having a hard time tolerating meat, I would whip up smoothies and add protein powder to them."
> —*Meghan*

- Rely on eggs for protein, vitamins, and minerals. See chapter 8 for tasty and nutritious egg recipes.

FROM THE RECIPE FILE

When your appetite is poor, consider drinking good nutrition in smoothies like Chocolate Banana Blast on page 225. Add whey protein or other protein powder and nut butter to boost calories and protein.

Your Exercise Routine Now

There are so many good reasons to exercise. When you're expecting, exercise has particular perks, including fewer aches and pains; less constipation, bloating, and swelling; improved energy level; stress reduction; and better sleep. Regular workouts during pregnancy can help you to cope better with labor and delivery, and they can also make it easier to get back in shape after your bundle of joy arrives.

Exercise reduces the risk for preeclampsia, a condition marked by elevated blood pressure, protein in your urine, and excessive water retention that may occur later in pregnancy. Regular workouts may help to prevent and to better manage gestational diabetes, the type of diabetes that first occurs during pregnancy, usually in the second trimester. It's tough to say exactly how much food you should add to your diet to account for regular exercise. The best measure of sufficient caloric intake during pregnancy is adequate weight gain.

As long as your health care provider approves, you should exercise on a regular basis. Women with uncomplicated pregnancies need a minimum of thirty minutes of moderate-intensity activity on most days of the week. There's no need to overexert yourself to reap the rewards of working out. It's best to spread the suggested amount of weekly exercise (two and a half hours) over many days.

You may already have a workout routine in place that you can continue, and as long as the activities you do are safe during pregnancy, you can keep up with it. However, you will probably have to modify your routine at some point. You'll tire more easily during pregnancy, so that forty-five-minute walk or the mile swim you've been doing all along could become challenging. As your pregnancy progresses, your ligaments and joints relax, too, as the body prepares itself for childbirth.

When you're just beginning to exercise on a regular basis, you might be more comfortable with programs that are specifically designed for pregnant women. No matter what activity you choose, always wear a bra that fits well and provides lots of support to help protect your breasts and make exercise comfortable. Invest in a new pair of comfortable sneakers and some loose-fitting workout gear, too.

Any Time Is a Good Time to Exercise

Even if you weren't active before you conceived, you can start at any point in your pregnancy, as long your health care provider says so. Now is not the time to take up a strenuous activity, however. In addition, there are some activities that you should put on hold until after delivery, even if you have been doing them for years (see "Do Not Try This at Home or Anywhere Else," on page 135).

Walking is beneficial for most pregnant women because it's easy on the joints and the muscles. Swimming works several muscle groups at once and helps you to sidestep injury because you're floating, and the water cools your body, allowing heat generated by working muscles to escape. Cycling on a stationary bike reduces the risk of falling, which increases as pregnancy progresses. Strength training relieves tension and makes stronger muscles, which helps to prevent some of the aches and pains common in pregnancy. Low-impact aerobic exercise is a good way to keep your heart and your lungs strong; as your pregnancy moves along, check out classes for pregnant women.

> ### Words of Motherly Wisdom
>
> "I swam when I was pregnant the second time around. I loved the feeling of weightlessness in the pool. I was in good shape going into delivery, and I bounced back faster than with my other pregnancies."
>
> —Meghan

Keep It Cool

A pregnant woman's body produces more heat because of a revved-up metabolism. In addition, working muscles generate heat that your body must release to maintain a normal (about 98.6°F) body temperature that's best for you and your baby.

Words of
Motherly Wisdom
"I'm a runner, and I thought
I'd be able to continue
during my third pregnancy,
but I could only run until
about the third month. I
was just so tired that I
chose sleep instead!"
—Erin

Overheating can be the result of exercising in a warm environment, such as a crowded aerobics room or gym, in hot and humid air, or in a combination of the two. Work out in cool, well-ventilated places, and wear loose-fitting clothing. Avoid hot tubs, saunas, and whirlpools to keep your body temperature normal.

Inadequate fluid intake is another cause of overheating. Dehydration reduces blood volume and decreases blood flow to your baby. Pregnant women need about 13 cups of fluid daily (from beverages and foods); pregnant exercisers will need more. Drink plenty of fluid before, during, and after working out. When your urine is plentiful and very light in color, you have a normal fluid balance. If it's dark and scanty, you need more fluid.

When Exercise Is Off-Limits

Exercise offers many benefits, but some pregnant women should not work out. According to the American College of Obstetricians and Gynecologists, women with the following, and other, conditions should avoid physical activity:

- Pregnancy-induced hypertension (high blood pressure)
- Preterm ruptured membranes (amniotic fluid leaks from the uterus)
- Preterm labor in the current pregnancy
- Insufficient cervix (the cervix dilates long before delivery)
- Persistent second- or third-trimester bleeding; the placenta is attached abnormally to the uterus or is loose or separating
- Severe anemia

If you're dedicated to fitness, being told to discontinue your workouts can come as a blow. However, pregnancy is relatively short. You may soon be back to exercising after your bundle of joy arrives.

Do Not Try This at Home or Anywhere Else!

Working out is good for you, but certain activities are out of the question when you're expecting because of the potential risks to you and your child. Any activity involving pressure changes that could deprive your baby of oxygen, and any sport with a high risk of falling or of abdominal trauma are inappropriate for pregnant women. Here's what *not* to do, even if you are a seasoned athlete or you've done these activities prior to pregnancy:

- Hiking at high altitudes or on rough, uneven terrain, and mountain climbing

- Anything with jumping or jarring motions, such as high-impact aerobics classes

- Certain yoga positions, including extreme backbends, inversions, and any positions that work your abdominal muscles or have you lie on your back

- Hot yoga or hot Pilates

- Off-road cycling

- Heavy lifting that involves straining

- Skydiving

- Surfing

- Kickboxing

- Boxing

- Scuba diving (snorkeling is okay)

- Downhill skiing or snowboarding (cross-country skiing is okay)

- Waterskiing

- Horseback riding

- Skateboarding

- Roller skating

- Ice skating

- Bike riding

- Contact sports such as ice hockey, soccer, touch or tackle football, lacrosse, and basketball

- Gymnastics

Words of Motherly Wisdom

"I found out I was pregnant with my first [child] one week after completing my first marathon. Even though I was very fit, I was shocked by how quickly I got winded once I was pregnant. I cut back to walking, and I am so glad that I did. It worked out great for me."

—Lisa

Know When to Say When

Stop exercising, and immediately call your doctor or other licensed health care professional, if you experience any of the following:

- Chest pain
- Vaginal bleeding
- Fluid leaking from the vagina
- Dizziness or feelings of faintness
- Headache

- Muscle weakness affecting balance
- Calf pain or swelling
- Contractions
- Increased shortness of breath, difficulty breathing

Mitigating Miscarriage

Miscarriage, the spontaneous loss of a baby during the first half of pregnancy, typically takes place in the first trimester. An estimated 10 to 15 percent of pregnancies end in miscarriage among women who know they are pregnant. Since many miscarriages occur long before a woman realizes that she's expecting, the actual miscarriage rate could be much higher.

Experts say that most first-trimester pregnancies end on their own because of chromosomal abnormalities in the embryo or fetus. Too many or too few chromosomes, the parts of cells that contain the genes, can result in devastating developmental difficulties and death. Second-trimester miscarriage (from thirteen to twenty weeks pregnant) is often caused by problems with the uterus or by a weakened cervix that dilates well before it should.

Nobody completely understands why most miscarriages happen, and, with the possible exception of alcohol intake, it's difficult to say exactly how nutrition influences miscarriage risk. However, research suggests that taking a daily multivitamin before pregnancy and throughout the first seven weeks after conception occurs may reduce pregnancy loss.

Age influences miscarriage risk, in part because chromosomal abnormalities are more common with the passage of time. Miscarriage rates are greater in women thirty-five and older, but the father's age may be a factor, too. Miscarriage risk is highest when the mother is thirty-five or older and her partner is forty or older. If you're in your mid-thirties and you're delaying pregnancy, you and your partner may realize the need to try to become pregnant sooner. If you are already pregnant, there's nothing you can do about your age, so there's no point in worrying. Instead, concentrate on how to bring your pregnancy to term. Start by seeking prenatal care as soon as possible and maintaining it throughout your pregnancy.

Diabetes, thyroid disease, PCOS, autoimmune disorders such as lupus, problems with the placenta, cervix, or uterus, and hormone problems can all cause miscarriage, too. Drug and alcohol use and cigarette smoking are also risk factors for pregnancy loss.

MOVING ON FROM MISCARRIAGE

If you've had a miscarriage, it might be comforting for you to know that it's often a one-time event. Counseling may help you cope with your grief of pregnancy loss. Later, when you do decide to try to get pregnant again, work closely with your health care provider to help improve your chances. Many women who have had one miscarriage often go on to have successful pregnancies.

THE SECOND TRIMESTER (WEEKS FOURTEEN TO TWENTY-SIX)

You'll probably feel your best during the second trimester; that's when a pregnant woman's energy typically returns. Many of the earlier effects of pregnancy subside during this trimester, including nausea, vomiting, and fatigue, but they do not all magically disappear once the fourteenth week begins.

As the second trimester of pregnancy proceeds, your baby's facial features are forming, and his heart is beating with regularity. Your baby is capable of making a fist with fully formed fingers and can even engage in thumb sucking, if so inclined. Tooth buds that will eventually become primary teeth have appeared, and it's possible to tell on ultrasound whether you're having a boy or a girl.

The second trimester is when your child's growth starts to take off. Bones, muscles, and organs become bigger and more developed. By the midpoint of your pregnancy—twenty weeks—your baby is about eight inches long. You might feel some turning, stretching, and kicking, starting around the sixteenth week. The heartbeat is stronger, so it's detectable with a stethoscope now. As the final trimester looms, an even more rapid development of the baby's brain and nervous system is on the horizon.

What to Eat Now

You need more food to fuel your baby's rapid growth. During the second trimester, that amounts to about 350 more calories a day compared to your prepregnancy and first-trimester energy needs. Your basic eating plan won't change dramatically, however. Consult the chart on page 59 ("Daily Portions from Each Food Group") to find out how much food to add from each of the food groups. If you have not done so, see chapter 3 to determine the appropriate MyPlate Prepregnancy plan for yourself, and make the wisest food choices for you and your child.

Even with the suggested guidelines, it's difficult to determine just how many calories a pregnant woman needs to gain the right amount of weight. That's because calorie needs are personal and can vary based on prepregnancy weight. As long as you're gaining adequate weight on a steady basis on a healthy diet, you're probably eating enough. Women who were very overweight before conceiving may need fewer calories on a daily basis.

Exceeding the recommended amount of weight during pregnancy may result in a bigger baby as well as more pregnancy pounds that are difficult to drop after delivery. Gaining too little weight is risky to the development of your child's full physical and mental potential. The proper amount of weight gain continues to be important after the second trimester, too; low weight gain during the third trimester is linked to a greater risk of preterm delivery.

Pregnancy Weight Gain

Eating more food means that you'll be putting on the pounds during the next nine months. If you have spent years trying to avoid extra body fat, gaining weight probably does not sit well with you, in spite of the excitement you feel about having a baby. However, gaining weight during pregnancy is for a very good cause. It may ease your mind to know how much weight to gain, why you must gain weight, and where it all goes.

The number of pounds you should put on when you're expecting depends on your prepregnancy body mass index (BMI) and on how many babies you're carrying. See chapter 1 to calculate your body mass index using your body weight prior to conception. The following list suggests how much weight to gain based on your preconception BMI.

If your BMI was . . .	Gain this much weight for a single baby	Gain this much weight for twins
Less than 18.5	28 to 40 pounds	n/a*
18.5 to 24.9	25 to 35 pounds	37 to 54 pounds
25.0 to 29.9	15 to 25 pounds	31 to 50 pounds
30.0 or greater	11 to 20 pounds	25 to 42 pounds

*No guidelines are available based on lack of sufficient research.

Where the Pregnancy Pounds Go

Your girth is expanding, and you'd like to know where all that extra weight is going! Here's an estimate:

Baby: $6^1/_2$ to 9 pounds

Placenta: $1^1/_2$ pounds

Amniotic fluid: 2 pounds

Breast enlargement: 1 to 3 pounds

Uterus enlargement: 2 pounds

Increased blood volume: 3 to 4 pounds

Increased fluid volume: 2 to 3 pounds

Fat stores and muscle development: 6 to 8 pounds

Total: 24 to $32^1/_2$ pounds

How Pregnancy Weight Gain Matters to Your Baby's Health

Birth weight is a good indicator of a baby's overall health at delivery and beyond. The size of your baby at birth is influenced largely by pregnancy weight gain. Putting on the recommended number of pounds based on your prepregnancy BMI helps your child achieve the best health possible.

Words of Motherly Wisdom

"Frankly, I was afraid I'd gain too much weight when I was pregnant. I am just not used to putting on the pounds. Educating myself about nutrition and pregnancy kept things in perspective for me."

—*Sarah*

Infants born to women who gain weight within the suggested range typically require fewer medical interventions after delivery, whereas children born to women who gain too little weight tend to be undersized and more likely to arrive before thirty-seven weeks (preterm birth). In addition to needing specialized medical care early in life, underweight babies (those weighing five pounds eight ounces or less) also run a greater risk of developing certain chronic conditions as young children and adults, including obesity, diabetes, high blood pressure, and heart disease.

Adequate weight gain also influences the mother's health during pregnancy. If you begin pregnancy at a healthy weight and put on more than thirty-five pounds, there's a greater chance of developing preeclampsia, a high blood pressure disorder, than if your weight gain is less than thirty-five pounds. Being overweight at conception *and* gaining more than the recommended number of pregnancy pounds increases the likelihood of gestational diabetes. Excess weight gain also increases your chances of a having a larger baby that requires cesarean delivery, and makes it harder to return to a healthy weight after the baby is born.

Starting Pregnancy with Extra Pounds

Beginning a pregnancy when you're overweight increases the odds of complications for both mother and child. The more overweight you are, the harder the pregnancy will be on you and your baby. If you're already pregnant, there's not much you can do now—or is there?

When researchers from the St. Louis University School of Medicine surveyed the results of the pregnancies of 120,000 obese women (defined as having a BMI of at least 30.0) who gained no more than fifteen pounds during pregnancy, they found that the risk of preeclampsia, cesarean delivery, and delivering larger babies decreased. Some of the women did deliver underweight babies, however. In a study of ninety-six obese women with gestational diabetes, researchers from the same medical school found that a combination of calorie restriction and exercise during pregnancy resulted in more babies of normal birth weight without any negative effects. Babies born to women who lost weight or maintained their weight while pregnant were more likely to be of normal size compared to the babies born to women who gained weight during the study.

If you're overweight and pregnant, do not put yourself on a diet. Ask your health care provider about your pregnancy-weight goals, and work with a RDN to develop an eating plan that's best for you.

Weight Gain: Timing Matters

When you gain weight during pregnancy is just as important as *how much* you gain. Perhaps you added just a few pounds to your frame during the first trimester, or none at all. It's a good idea to gain weight on a steady basis from the second trimester to delivery day.

Once the first trimester has passed, plan to add a pound or so each week, or about four pounds per month. Overweight women (those starting pregnancy at a BMI of 25.0 or above) should add about half a pound weekly, or about two pounds per month.

You might not gain weight according to the guidelines. For example, women who still experience some nausea and vomiting during the second trimester may gain

> ### Words of Motherly Wisdom
>
> "I was overweight when I become pregnant. I figured there was nothing I could do but eat the best way possible from then on, which is what I did with the help of my dietitian. I had a healthy baby boy!"
> —Amy

slightly less weight until they feel better. If you consistently gain too little or too much weight from one doctor's visit to the next, it can be a sign that your diet should be adjusted or that you have another problem.

If you're gaining weight too quickly, review the suggested eating pattern in your MyPlate Pregnancy Plan and see how closely you're sticking to it. You may need to adjust portion sizes; choose foods with less fat and/or added sugar, like grilled chicken instead of fried, 1% low-fat milk instead of whole, and plain oatmeal instead of the sugary flavored kind. Check your diet for excessively salty foods, such as canned soups and other processed and fast foods, including pizza, to see whether sodium is to blame for water retention that can increase the number on the scale. Women who have excessive weight gain during pregnancy shouldn't attempt to lose what they have put on, but they should try to bring their rate of gain within a healthy range.

Inadequate weight gain during pregnancy is most likely due to not eating enough. You may need to recalculate your calorie needs according to MyPlate, and be sure to include all of the recommended servings every day. Persistent nausea and vomiting, which can last for an entire pregnancy, may be another reason for inadequate calorie intake. Women who gain too much weight or not enough weight for any reason during their pregnancies would benefit from the advice of an RDN.

Gestational Diabetes

Around the twenty-fourth week of your pregnancy, you should have a blood test for gestational diabetes mellitus (GDM). GDM is the form of diabetes that occurs for the first time when a woman is pregnant. See chapter 7 for details about GDM and testing for GDM.

REALITY CHECK: MORE THAN A BABY BUMP

Celebrities and others who appear to have just a baby bump and no other pregnancy weight gain get a lot of attention, but they may not be eating enough. Don't follow in their footsteps. Intentionally restricting calories to keep weight gain low during pregnancy can harm your baby's growth and development.

Managing Pregnancy Cravings

Once the first trimester is over, your appetite may return, and with a vengeance! You've probably heard tales of partners being dispatched at all hours to search for a certain brand of bacon double cheeseburger or rocky road ice cream to quell an expectant mother's desire. Now you're the one with the pregnancy cravings.

Intense longings for salty chips, stuffed-crust pizza, and double chocolate chip cookies are most likely being driven by pregnancy hormones. Craving certain foods and eating them can also be how you comfort yourself when you're tired or crabby.

Words of Motherly Wisdom

"After having avoided meat for nearly seven years, I had unbelievable and undeniable cravings for red meat during my first pregnancy. I could not get enough! But my other two pregnancies didn't have the same effect. In fact, with my third, I had very little appetite—at least at first."

—*Lisa*

KEEP CRAVINGS SAFE

No matter how strong the craving is, don't give in to eating raw or undercooked seafood (including sushi and sashimi), raw meat, or raw eggs; unpasteurized juice, unpasteurized milk, or foods made from unpasteurized milk, including Brie, feta, Camembert, Roquefort, and Mexican-style cheeses; raw sprouts, including alfalfa, clover, and radish; certain herbal teas not sold in the supermarket; and alcohol. These foods, and others, are more likely to make you sick during pregnancy or to endanger the growth and development of your baby. See chapter 6 for more on food safety.

Eating too much of any food, healthy or otherwise, during pregnancy may lead to excessive weight gain that boosts the risk for complications, including gestational diabetes and high blood pressure. Fast food, snacks, and sugary soft drinks may replace foods that offer more nutrition for you and your baby. You do not have to give up snacking or eating the foods you crave, but you need to count the calories from these and other snacks as part of your daily calorie budget. Try to control pregnancy cravings using the following simple strategies:

- Eat on a regular basis to prevent intense hunger that can trigger cravings.

- Make sure that your meals include a balance of protein, carbohydrates, and healthy fat.

- Know that indulging is OK, in small amounts. For example, when you can't resist chips, choose a one-ounce bag of the baked variety instead of a large bag of the fried kind. Or mindfully munch a fun-size candy bar instead of gobbling a whole one, which may be enough to satisfy an urge.

- Consider your hunger level. Maybe you just need a short break to relieve stress, and not food.

When cravings strike before, during, or after pregnancy, reach for these healthier options:

Crunchy. Instead of regular snack chips, try chips made from toasted whole-wheat pita bread with melted grated Parmesan cheese; an ounce of nuts or sunflower seeds; low-fat popcorn; an ounce of reduced-fat cheese, such as cheddar, and six whole-grain crackers; ten small whole-grain pretzels topped with a tablespoon of almond or peanut butter; a quarter cup of trail mix (equal parts whole-grain cereal, chopped nuts, dried fruit, sunflower seeds, and miniature chocolate chips); or raw carrots or celery.

Creamy. Instead of a big bowl of ice cream, reach for a small bowl of sorbet, gelato, or frozen yogurt; 8 ounces of low-fat vanilla, coffee, or fruit-flavored yogurt; or a smoothie made with fruit and yogurt.

Chocolate. Enjoy chocolate pudding prepared with low-fat milk; a 100-calorie frozen fudge bar; hot chocolate or chocolate milk made with low-fat milk; chocolate-dipped strawberries or dried fruit; or a choco-banana frappe made with a cup of low-fat chocolate milk, one medium banana, and two ice cubes.

Sweet. Skip the pastry and have one of these healthier options: two graham crackers spread with low-fat cream cheese and strawberry jam; half a whole-wheat bagel topped with peanut butter and drizzled with honey; a piece of whole-grain toast spread with half a cup of part-skim ricotta cheese and sprinkled with a quarter teaspoon of sugar and a pinch of ground cinnamon; angel food cake drizzled with chocolate or coffee sauce; frozen pops made with 100 percent orange juice; sherbet; frozen fruit; or dried fruit.

PICA: CRAVINGS GONE WRONG

Pica is the term for the cravings that some pregnant women have for nonfood items, including dirt, clay, paper, and even paint chips. No one knows the exact cause of pica, but it may be a sign of iron and zinc deficiencies in the diet. Expectant mothers may also get the urge to eat raw flour or cornstarch, which, despite being food items, are problematic in large amounts; too much can lead to blocked bowels and can replace essential nutrients in the diet by causing feelings of fullness. If you feel compelled to consume nonfood items, including ice, report such cravings to your health care provider immediately.

Coping with Stress

Stress is part of our daily lives. Some stress is considered beneficial because it motivates us to get things done. Persistent, severe stress is not good, however, especially when you're pregnant. Divorce, the death of a loved one, job loss, worry about your relationship with your baby's father, or financial woes are all sources of stress that can be detrimental to you and your child during pregnancy.

High levels of ongoing stress can result in fatigue, sleeplessness, poor appetite, and headaches, among other side effects. In some cases, severe stress boosts the risk of preterm birth.

Words of Motherly Wisdom

"Even though your life is stressful, once you get pregnant, you have to take time for yourself to relax. You and your baby need it."

—*Meghan*

Poor nutrition makes it more difficult to deal with stress, whether you're pregnant or not. Eating a healthy diet and taking a multivitamin every day can provide some of the stamina you need to deal with constant stress. Regular physical activity, as long as it has been approved by your doctor, relieves stress, too.

Preeclampsia

Although relatively uncommon, preeclampsia is a potentially dangerous condition that can develop quickly in the second trimester or later in pregnancy. Preeclampsia is marked by elevated blood pressure, swelling due to fluid retention, and abnormal kidney function that results in protein spilling into the urine. See chapter 7 for details about preeclampsia.

Fighting Food Allergies

A food allergy is an overreaction to the proteins in foods called *allergens.* When you have a food allergy, the body's immune system interprets harmless food allergens as invaders and sets in motion a cascade of events to get rid of the threat. Food allergies can cause problems such as eczema, as well as life-threatening reactions. The allergens in foods cannot be destroyed by cooking or through digestion.

Food allergies are frightening, so you want to do everything possible to prevent your child from becoming allergic to milk, eggs, peanuts, tree nuts (such as walnuts and almonds), fish, shellfish, soy, or wheat—the foods that account for 90 percent of all food-allergic reactions. If you, your partner, or one of your children has a food allergy, your future children are more prone to having one, too.

You may have heard that it's possible to reduce the risk of food allergy in your child by avoiding highly allergenic foods during pregnancy or breastfeeding. Current thinking on the topic says otherwise, however. Even if your baby is at higher risk of developing food allergy, experts say eating a balanced diet that includes all foods during pregnancy and breastfeeding is the best course. Talk to your doctor about your concerns.

Exclusively breastfeeding your child for at least four and up to six months is helpful for reducing food allergy. If you're formula feeding and you have a baby at high risk of food allergy, talk to your pediatrician about using a hydrolyzed infant formula. Also, it's OK to start feeding your child solid foods between four and six months of age, including early exposure to potential allergens, such as peanut products like thinned peanut butter, to prevent the development of food allergy. However, if your child has moderate to severe eczema, or egg allergy, or both, discuss how and when you should introduce potentially allergenic foods, such as peanuts, with your doctor.

ALLERGY OR INTOLERANCE?

An intolerance to a certain food is sometimes misinterpreted as a food allergy. For example, lactose intolerance, the inability of the body to break down lactose, the natural carbohydrate in milk, is not a milk allergy because it does not involve the immune system. The symptoms of lactose intolerance, including gas, bloating, and diarrhea, are uncomfortable, but they are fleeting and don't cause lasting harm. Ask your doctor or an allergist about any adverse reactions you have to a food to be sure of the difference between a food allergy and food intolerance.

Exercise During the Second Trimester: Keep Moving

By the second trimester, you might be feeling energetic again. Take advantage of this renewed get-up-and-go and start working out, if you haven't been doing so already. As always, ask your doctor what type of physical activity is best for you, even if you have been exercising since the beginning of your pregnancy. Exercise can be dangerous for women with pregnancy-induced high blood pressure or other conditions. Make sure you're eating the right amount of food to keep your weight gain on track.

For the previous thirteen weeks, your blood levels of pregnancy hormones, particularly progesterone, have been on the rise. That's beneficial, because progesterone preps your body to expand in order to accommodate a growing child and for childbirth. However, the effects of progesterone have a downside because they make pregnant women more prone to injury. Avoid jerky, bouncy, or high-impact motions to keep from hurting yourself. See page 135 for activities to avoid during pregnancy.

Carrying extra pounds causes your body to work harder, even when you're doing the same amount of exercise to which you're accustomed. The additional weight in your front shifts your center of gravity, stressing the joints and the muscles in your lower back and pelvis. As the second trimester comes to a close, you may experience more back pain and become prone to losing your balance. You might feel more confident with exercise programs that are designed for pregnant women, including yoga and aerobics.

> ### Words of Motherly Wisdom
>
> "I'm in my second trimester now. I wear a heart-rate monitor when I work out because I've been told to keep my heart rate under 140 beats per minute."
>
> —Kasie

Your growing uterus will probably press on your diaphragm, making it harder to take the deep breaths you need when you're working out. If you're able to carry on a normal conversation during exercise, then you are within an acceptable range for exertion. Swimming and water aerobics will reduce the pressure on your diaphragm.

Do not exercise while lying flat on your back now. Lying down compresses a large blood vessel called the *vena cava*. The vena cava shuttles blood to and from the heart, so pressing on it could cause a sudden drop in blood pressure, dizziness, or a loss of consciousness. Circulation of blood through the body slows down with weight gain, so you are more likely to retain fluid in your legs and ankles.

Although it's important to be careful when you're working out, don't be put off from regular physical activity. You're doing yourself and your baby a big favor when you exercise on most days of the week. Being in shape before delivery usually means a faster return to fitness after giving birth.

THE THIRD TRIMESTER (WEEKS TWENTY-SEVEN TO FORTY)

You're in the home stretch! In just a short while, your baby will make her debut. Your child is really growing now. From the start of the third trimester to delivery day (about thirteen weeks), her body weight will double, and your weight gain will largely reflect that growth as the baby adds fat and accumulates nutrients such as calcium and iron. Whether you plan on nursing your child or not, your breasts are counting on it. You may have noticed a recent expansion as they prepare to produce milk.

Words of Motherly Wisdom

"With all three of my kids, I always found the last trimester to be both nerve-wracking and exciting. I couldn't wait to see my new baby!"
—*Shana*

The baby's organs, most notably the brain and the lungs, continue to mature to handle life outside the womb. Your baby's brain development is rapid from about the twenty-fourth week on, and her eyes are preparing to take in the world very soon. By birth, your child will probably measure nineteen to twenty-one inches from head to toe. Babies can either have a full head of hair or be completely bald when they arrive.

A child is considered full-term at thirty-seven weeks, but the goal is forty weeks. Toward the end of your pregnancy, you should be checking in with your health care provider on a weekly basis (more often if you're having more than one baby) to monitor your health and your baby's health.

THIRD-TRIMESTER TO-DO LIST

- Discuss your birth plan with the doctor or certified nurse-midwife who will deliver your baby.

- Take a prenatal class to help ease delivery-day jitters.

- Find a pediatrician. Check with your insurance company, get advice from friends, or ask your hospital for a referral. Meet with your pediatrician before you deliver, if possible.

- Get a group B strep culture. Some women carry strep B, a normally harmless bacteria that can cause infection in newborns. Women who test positive should receive antibiotics during labor.

- Buy a car seat and make sure it's properly installed. You won't be allowed to leave the hospital without one.

- Prepare to feed. If you're going to breastfeed, purchase a breast pump and learn how to use it now. Make sure you have a supply of comfortable clothes you can easily nurse in, as well as nursing bras and nursing pads. All parents should stock up on bottles and nipples. Even if you plan to breastfeed, you may eventually want to pump milk so that someone other than you can feed your child. If you're not planning to breastfeed, buy infant formula, and learn how to make it correctly according to manufacturer's directions.

What to Eat Now

It's as important as ever to continue taking a daily multivitamin and other supplements, such as extra iron and calcium, as needed.

Your calorie needs in the third trimester are the highest they'll be during pregnancy. The irony is that you need to eat more—about 450 additional calories than your daily prepregnancy needs—but as your due date approaches, you may find it increasingly difficult to include all that food. Your expanding uterus and the baby it carries crowds your stomach during the third trimester. A cramped abdominal area is probably to blame for heartburn, too. Try dividing up your daily calorie allowance into six small, nourishing meals. Read more about handling heartburn in chapter 7.

Toward the end of the trimester, you might not be sleeping as well because it can be difficult to get comfortable. Healthy eating can't cure your fatigue, but it certainly can help. Eat more frequently to keep your energy level as high as possible. Another irritation will be pressure on your bladder, which means that you'll probably get up a few times a night to pee and will also need to go frequently during the day. Restricting fluid intake won't help matters, however. Try lying on your side to take the stress off your kidneys, and always empty your bladder before retiring for the night.

Your child's brain size increases significantly from about the twenty-fourth week of pregnancy to the fortieth. It's especially important to include the nutrients your child needs to support brain development, including protein, DHA, and choline, which are discussed in detail in chapter 2.

FROM THE RECIPE FILE

Spinach, Red Bell Pepper, and Cheese Cups (page 240) are perfect for when you can't eat a lot of food all at once, and they are packed with choline.

Exercise During the Third Trimester: Stay Safe

Your body is gearing up for delivery, so it's probably more limber than you think. It's especially important to pay attention to how you feel during exercise. Don't push yourself! It's not worth risking injury.

By the end of the pregnancy, you probably won't be doing much more than walking, swimming, or prenatal exercise classes, because everything else might be too uncomfortable, given your size and the change in your center of gravity. Nevertheless, many women work out right up until delivery day. Just remember to take it at your own pace, and be sure to eat enough and drink enough fluids.

Prepare Your Kitchen

You might not know whether you're having a boy or a girl, but one thing is for sure: you'll be busy after the baby is born, and you won't have time to prepare complicated meals. Eating properly after delivery is key to bouncing back from nine months of pregnancy and childbirth, however. It's especially important for breast-feeding mothers. Avoid "flying by the seat of your pants" once the baby arrives. Stock your

Words of Motherly Wisdom

"I bought a separate freezer when I was pregnant and did a lot of food preparation so that I'd have something in reserve."

—Janice

cupboards, refrigerator, and freezer with foods now to get you through the first few months with a minimum of fuss.

Load up on no-salt-added canned and frozen foods that are easy to prepare in a pinch, including fruits, vegetables, canned and pouched salmon and tuna, and beans (chickpeas, black beans, and edamame). Purchase lean meat, poultry, and seafood, such as bags of frozen shrimp, to freeze, and label each package with the amount of food it contains and the date you put it in the freezer. Make sure you have condiments on hand, including balsamic and red wine vinegars, olive and canola oils, jelly or jam, ketchup, mayonnaise, mustard, salad dressing, and any others that you enjoy. Purchase boxes of whole-grain cereal, pasta, whole grains (such as quick-cooking brown rice, wild rice, quinoa, and freekeh), and nuts and nut butters (peanut, almond, or sunflower seed). Add frozen whole-wheat pizza crusts to your kitchen survival grocery list.

> ### Words of Motherly Wisdom
>
> "I live in an area where a lot of the local take-out and delivery restaurants serve healthy cuisine, such as Japanese, Thai, and Middle Eastern, so I kept those menus close by during the months after my son was born."
>
> —Dina

Begin preparing meals, such as large batches of casseroles, lasagnas, stews, and soups, to freeze. If space is tight, consider buying a chest freezer. Label each gallon-size container or resealable storage bag (which are great because you can freeze them lying flat and they don't take up as much room, and you're not tying up all of your heavy-duty plastic containers) with the date of preparation.

FROM THE RECIPE FILE

Soups and stews freeze well, and so does the base of Cauliflower Crust Personal Pizza with Mushrooms, Olives, and Goat Cheese (page 282). Make the crust ahead of time, freeze, and finish preparing the pizza when you like.

Decision Time: How Will You Feed Your Baby?

You've decorated the baby's room and have even decided on a name for your impending arrival. Have you given much thought to how you'll feed your baby?

Breast milk is one of nature's most perfectly designed foods and, as such, is considered the best choice for newborns and infants. Several health organizations, including the American Academy of Pediatrics (AAP), recommend breastfeeding exclusively for at least six months, and preferably for at least twelve months and even longer, along with other foods. Don't let that time frame scare you; any amount of nursing is beneficial to your baby and to you.

Perhaps you have been unsuccessful at breastfeeding in the past. That doesn't mean you'll have trouble this time around. If you have other children and you've never nursed before, give it a try. You can always start with breastfeeding your baby and switch to infant formula, but it usually doesn't happen the other way around, at least not after the first few days following delivery have passed (although it's not impossible). Of course, it's not always possible to breastfeed, even if you're willing.

Words of Motherly Wisdom

"I was nervous about nursing because my mother never did, and a lot of friends had no experience with it, so I didn't know whom I could turn to for advice. Still, I tried it, and it worked out great for me and my children."

—*Shana*

If you're going back to work in a few months and you think that breastfeeding is out of the question, you may be interested to know that there are many ways to make breastfeeding succeed when you are away from your baby for hours at a time, such as pumping breast milk that your baby takes from a bottle from someone else, and breastfeeding your baby when you're with him. Even if you nurse your child for a short time before returning to work, and then switch the feedings to infant formula, you have done your baby a world of good.

Breastfeeding: What's in It for You and Your Child

Breast milk is easily digested, and it contains all the nutrients a baby needs for the first six months of life. Babies who nurse benefit in numerous ways from breast milk's protective qualities. The health benefits of breastfeeding are both short-term and long-lasting for you and your child.

Breastfeeding helps to boost a baby's immune system and possibly reduces the risk of ear infections and infections in the digestive and upper respiratory tracts. It may also lessen the likelihood of asthma and allergies, type 1 diabetes, and leukemia and lymphoma in children. According to the AAP, research shows that breastfeeding for at least four months after birth reduces the prevalence of celiac disease in infants when they are first fed gluten-containing foods, such as a wheat-based cereal. Breastfed babies may be less likely to become overweight later in life, too.

Breast milk contains DHA, which helps to promote brain development and possibly boost intelligence. However, mom's diet must include 200 to 300 mg of DHA daily so that baby can benefit. See chapter 3 for more on DHA. If breast milk has a fault, it is that it's low in vitamin D. The AAP recommends that all babies, including those who are exclusively breastfed, consume at least 400 IU of vitamin D as dietary supplements (drops) every day beginning in the first days of life to help prevent rickets, a bone-weakening disease. Infants get adequate vitamin D in infant formula.

Besides being economical and convenient, breastfeeding can be an amazing and rewarding experience for a woman and her child. Nursing aids in your body's ability to return to its prepregnancy state faster. Breastfeeding triggers the production of hormones that cause your uterus to contract, making it smaller and firmer. Nursing a child might also lower the risk of premenopausal breast cancer, and of ovarian cancer, and may help women avoid type 2 diabetes if they did not have gestational diabetes.

Nervous About Nursing?

You may be wondering if you'll be able to breastfeed successfully. It's normal to be nervous about breastfeeding, especially with your first child, if you're having more than one baby at a time, or if you expect to deliver your baby before thirty-seven weeks. Speak with friends and family who have been successful at nursing, or talk with your certified nurse-midwife, obstetrician, nurse practitioner, or a lactation consultant. Take a breastfeeding class to learn the basics.

Who Should Not Breastfeed?

Breastfeeding is recommended for nearly all mothers and their children, including mothers of multiple babies. However, there are those who should not nurse, including the following:

- Women with HIV (human immunodeficiency virus, the virus that causes AIDS), because they can pass the virus to their babies in their breast milk

- Women taking antiretroviral medications

- Women with untreated tuberculosis

- Women who are taking drugs for cancer treatment, including radioactive compounds

- Women who are using or dependent upon an illicit (illegal) drug

- Women whose babies have galactosemia, a rare genetic disorder that impedes a baby's ability to process the carbohydrates in breast milk (and dairy-based formula). Newborn screening tests detect most babies with galactosemia soon after birth.

Women who have chronic health conditions that are controlled with medication (including prescription drugs, over-the-counter drugs, and herbal supplements) should check with their doctors before breastfeeding. Some medications and dietary supplements pose a risk to breastfeeding babies.

Formula Feeding

Women choose formula for a number of reasons, including physical or medical reasons or because they plan on returning to work soon after delivering and don't think it will be convenient or possible to pump breast milk at the office. Other mothers want to share the feeding responsibility, and they think that formula feeding makes the best sense for all involved.

The makers of infant formula strive to come as close as possible to duplicating the composition of human milk, and they do a good job of it. Once you've decided on infant formula, the question becomes which type to use. Formulas based on cow's milk are a fine choice for most babies, unless they have an intolerance or a milk allergy. Make sure the formula you pick is fortified with iron so that your baby receives the right amount of this vital nutrient. Choose a formula that is also fortified with the healthy fats DHA and arachadonic acid (AA). Nutrition experts say that you should choose an infant formula with a DHA level of at least 0.2 percent of the total fatty acids, and the level of AA should not be lower than that of DHA. If the levels of DHA and AA are not listed on the infant formula label, contact the manufacturer to find out.

The final decision about formula is what form to use. Infant formula comes as ready-to-feed, as concentrated liquid, or as powder. Powdered formulas are generally the least expensive, but they also require the most work to prepare. Breastfeeding mothers who supplement their milk supply with powdered infant formula can easily mix the formula they need from powder, without waste. Never make infant formula from your own "recipe." See chapter 5 for more on infant formula.

REALITY CHECK: GUILT-FREE FEEDING CHOICES

After hearing about all the wonders of breast milk, you may be worried or feel guilty about giving your child infant formula. Don't be. Many generations have been raised on infant formula, which just keeps improving in quality as researchers discover more ways to mimic the components of breast milk. You should never feel shame about a choice that works best for you and your family.

A LOOK AT WHAT'S AHEAD

This chapter highlighted the healthy lifestyle habits that will serve you well during each stage of pregnancy. There's no need to stop taking such good care of yourself after delivery day, and every reason to keep up the good work, especially if there are more children in your future. The next chapter helps you to navigate the "fourth trimester," when your body makes its way back to its nonpregnant self.

5

The Fourth Trimester: After the Baby Arrives

Congratulations on the birth of your baby! For the last nine months, and possibly longer, you've worked hard caring for yourself and your developing child. Now that delivery day has come and gone, you're on to the next phase of parenthood: the postpartum (after pregnancy) months, often referred to as the "fourth trimester."

During the fourth trimester, your body returns to its nonpregnant state. This early postpartum period is also when you and your family start adjusting to life with an infant and establish routines that work best for you.

You were transformed during pregnancy, seemingly stretched to the limit as your due date approached. A long delivery may have left you worn out. After all, they don't call it labor for nothing! Right now, you may be sore, achy, and really tired.

If you had a cesarean delivery, you're recovering from the additional stress of surgery. You may also have some swelling that has yet to disappear. Postdelivery puffiness is even more likely with cesarean deliveries because of the intravenous fluids you received during the procedure. Don't worry—in a few days, you should start to lose the extra fluid you're carrying. Significant swelling, however, can signal a serious problem, such as a blood clot. If you're excessively puffy and have pain or swelling that's worse on one side of the body, let your health care provider know immediately.

Swollen breasts are par for the course. Breast milk production revs up about two to five days after your baby is born. Mothers who have decided to use infant formula to feed their baby can apply cold compresses on their breasts to limit milk production. For breastfeeding women, breast engorgement is avoidable by nursing as often as your child wants to eat and by expressing extra milk with a breast pump when you're separated from your baby for long periods. Breast milk can be frozen or refrigerated for future use.

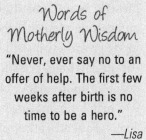

Words of Motherly Wisdom

"Never, ever say no to an offer of help. The first few weeks after birth is no time to be a hero."

—*Lisa*

Expect some vaginal bleeding for up to six weeks after delivery. This is a normal process as the body rids itself of uterine tissue it no longer needs. Although mild bleeding during this time is OK, fever and pain in the abdominal area are not. You may feel somewhat crampy at times, especially if you breastfeed, as your uterus shrinks back to its normal size, a process that can take months to complete.

POSTPARTUM APPOINTMENTS

If the postpartum period is problem-free for you, the next visit you'll have with your health care professional should be four to six weeks after delivery—probably sooner if you had a cesarean delivery or pregnancy complications. The appointment should include a thorough physical exam. Use the visit to discuss any aspect of your well-being that you want to address, including how you're adjusting emotionally to your new role as a parent; how the new baby is affecting your relationship with your spouse or partner; your fatigue level; and when you can start exercising again and how much physical activity is right for you.

WHAT YOU SHOULD EAT NOW

Mothers with newborn babies constantly battle exhaustion. A healthy lifestyle is no substitute for getting enough shut-eye, but eating right and getting regular physical activity lessen fatigue and stress. Nutritious foods provide you with the energy to cope with an infant who seems to eat all day long, cries for no reason for hours at a time, and requires a dozen or more diaper changes a day. In addition to tending a newborn, you may be managing other children, a household, or a job.

A balanced eating plan will help your body to heal. To make your recovery go more smoothly, finish taking the remainder of your prescription prenatal vitamins along with other additional supplements you may need, such as calcium and DHA. When your prenatal vitamins run out, substitute a daily multivitamin. See more on choosing a multivitamin in chapter 1.

After a few weeks, you'll probably start yearning to wear your pre-baby clothes. Hold off on trying to fit into your "before" jeans for at least six weeks after delivery because doing so any sooner may require a low-calorie diet. Instead, follow a balanced eating plan with a minimum of 1,800 calories (nursing mothers need more calories; see below) to allow your body to recover from nine months of pregnancy and from childbirth. Rely on a MyPlate plan, discussed in chapter 3, to guide you to safe weight loss. Do not skip meals, especially breakfast, even if you have to eat them in stages and not all at once while sitting down.

Research suggests that it's harder to take off pregnancy weight after twelve months have passed. There's no rush, but do try to shed pregnancy pounds during the first year after delivery by getting some physical activity on most days of the week and by following an eating pattern that

Words of Motherly Wisdom

"The night after coming home from the hospital with my first baby, I was so excited to have my favorite broccoli and onion pizza, because most of what I had read said that my diet wouldn't affect my baby while breastfeeding. What a mistake! Neither one of us slept the entire night. His stomach was so upset!"

—Kasie

provides the right amount of food for weight loss. Don't cut calories by too much if you're breastfeeding.

FROM THE RECIPE FILE

Craving comfort? Dig into Shepherd's Pie (page 270).
It's easy to make and packed with protein and vegetables.
Plus, you'll probably have leftovers for another meal!

WHAT TO EAT WHEN YOU'RE BREASTFEEDING

Breastfeeding moms need 330 more calories every day than they do when not pregnant; that's about the amount suggested during the second trimester of pregnancy. If you nurse for more than six months, increase your daily intake by 400 calories a day. Follow the MyPlate Postpregnancy Plan, and take a daily multivitamin so that you and your baby get the nutrients you both need.

Breastfeeding women require 200 to 300 milligrams (mg) of DHA every day to help maximize the baby's brain and visual development. Getting enough omega-3 fats, particularly DHA, can be difficult if you don't include fish or foods fortified with DHA, such as eggs. (See chapter 2 for more on DHA.) You should consider taking DHA supplements if your diet does not provide enough of this important fat.

Although breast milk is considered the perfect food for babies, it lacks adequate vitamin D to protect their growing bones. Vitamin D is essential to the movement of calcium into and out of the bones, and it's particularly powerful for preventing rickets, which causes soft, weak bones in children. Vitamin D production in the body starts in skin that's been exposed to strong sunlight and finishes in the liver and kidneys. Technically, your child's body can make all of the vitamin D it needs. However, it's unlikely that your infant will produce adequate vitamin D, because most babies don't, and shouldn't, spend enough time in the sunlight to stimulate vitamin D production. That's why the American Academy of Pediatrics recommends 400 international units (IU) of supplemental vitamin D every day for breastfed infants, beginning in the first days of life. Your pediatrician should prescribe a vitamin D supplement as drops for your child. Infant formula contains adequate vitamin D.

Now that you're finished with pregnancy, you'd probably like to go back to having a glass of wine or a cocktail or two when you're out to dinner. An occasional drink is probably OK during breastfeeding, but it's not advisable to make it a habit. Alcohol gets into breast milk. It can slow the development of your child's motor skills, which influences activities like walking and grabbing large objects. Beer, wine, and hard liquor can also interfere with your baby's ability to get milk from you during nursing. Alcohol inhibits the production of oxytocin, a hormone that encourages the flow of breast milk. If you do try breastfeeding your child while alcohol is active in your system, don't be surprised if you have difficulty "letting down," or getting the milk to flow easily. Wait at least two hours after your last drink to breastfeed for the alcohol to clear out of your system so that you reduce the risk of exposing your child to alcohol.

Be aware that nicotine and other harmful chemicals in cigarettes also make their way into breast milk. Moreover, smoking around a newborn raises the risk of sudden infant death syndrome (SIDS). Secondhand smoke is dangerous for newborns, young children, and everyone else, so if you quit smoking while you were pregnant, do your best to stay away from tobacco, e-cigarettes, and hookah.

Don't rely too heavily on caffeine for an energy boost. Caffeine may provide the jolt you need to keep going as the mother of a newborn, but keep in mind that it will have the same effect on your child, maybe even more so. Babies can't process caffeine as quickly as adults, so consuming it can leave you with a child who is irritable and has difficulty settling down to go to sleep, perhaps just when you're completely worn out and looking forward to some rest. For your sake and the baby's, when you're breastfeeding, limit the caffeine you consume from coffee, tea, and other caffeine-containing beverages and foods to under 300 mg a day. See chapter 2 for more on caffeine.

NO RECIPE REQUIRED: MAKE MEALS IN MINUTES

You're a busy mom with little time to feed yourself. The following simple meals might not be your idea of gourmet food, but they are easy-to-assemble solutions that are in keeping with different eating styles and the MyPlate eating plans. You can make some of these earlier in the day and grab them to eat when you sit down to breastfeed your child, dash out of the house to do errands, or have a few minutes to yourself. See chapter 8 for more ideas for healthy meals, snacks, and desserts.

Breakfast/Lunch Ideas

- Top a 2-ounce whole-wheat bagel with 2 tablespoons peanut butter, almond butter, or sunflower seed butter. Serve with 1 cup 1% low-fat milk or fortified soy milk, and fruit.

- Scramble 2 eggs, and divide equally between a 7-inch whole-wheat pita round that's been cut in half. Add salsa, a handful of spinach, and $1/4$ cup shredded reduced-fat cheese, if desired. Pair with 1 cup milk or fortified soy milk.

- Scramble 2 eggs with $1/4$ cup diced mushrooms and $1/4$ cup shredded reduced-fat cheddar cheese. Serve with 2 slices whole-wheat toast and jam and fruit.

- Pair 1 hard-cooked egg, 1 cup low-fat yogurt, 1 slice whole-grain toast, and fruit.

- Halve a cantaloupe or honeydew melon, remove the seeds, and fill with 1 cup cottage cheese or low-fat vanilla or plain yogurt. Serve with a whole-wheat roll.

- Spread 2 slices whole-grain bread with 2 tablespoons sunflower seed butter, and top with 1 small banana, sliced, or 2 tablespoons raisins.

Lunch/Dinner Ideas

- Microwave a medium white potato. Scoop out the insides and mix with 1 cup cottage cheese. Return the filling to the potato skins and warm in the microwave. Add a green salad.

- Spread 1 small whole-wheat pita round with tomato sauce, and top with sliced part-skim mozzarella cheese. Broil until cheese melts. Serve with 1 cup 100% orange juice.

- Make a quick quesadilla using two whole-wheat 7-inch sandwich wraps, 2 ounces chopped leftover chicken, and 1 ounce Monterey Jack cheese. Grill in a skillet. Enjoy with fruit.

- In a bowl, layer 1 cup cooked whole-grain couscous, 1 cup cooked vegetables, and 4 ounces cooked leftover salmon, or canned or pouched salmon.

- Arrange 4 ounces canned, drained tuna, 10 whole-grain crackers, and sliced red bell pepper, and enjoy.

- Mix 1 cup canned reduced-sodium lentil soup and 1 cup cooked pasta or other leftover cooked grain such as farro, brown rice, freekeh, or quinoa. Serve with 1 cup milk or fortified soy milk and fruit.

- Combine 1 cup canned white beans, drained, with 1 tablespoon olive oil and 4 ounces peeled and clean raw shrimp in a skillet. Cook until shrimp are pink. Serve with fruit or vegetables.

- Stir-fry $1/2$ pound ground skinless turkey breast meat or 95 percent lean ground beef with chopped onions and $1/2$ teaspoon ground cumin. Spoon cooked meat onto 2 whole-wheat tortillas along with chopped tomato, lettuce, and low-fat sour cream or plain Greek yogurt. (This dish serves two.) Serve with fruit or vegetables.

- Coat 4 ounces thinly sliced chicken breasts or tenders with flour. Heat 1 tablespoon olive oil in a medium skillet over medium heat. Cook chicken for about two minutes on each side. Pile onto a whole-wheat sandwich bun and garnish with tomato and lettuce. Serve with 1 cup milk and a piece of fruit.

- Quick fried rice: Heat 2 teaspoons canola oil in a medium skillet. Add 1 cup cold cooked white or brown rice, $1/4$ cup chopped onion, $1/4$ cup cooked peas or diced carrots or both, and 2 beaten eggs. Toss the entire mixture until the egg is cooked. Season with a dash of low-sodium soy sauce. Serve with fresh fruit.

- Place 4 ounces cooked shrimp, canned tuna, cooked salmon, cottage cheese, or tofu, on top of 2 cups chopped leafy greens and $1/2$ cup grape tomatoes. Top with a mixture of 2 teaspoons olive oil and balsamic vinegar. Serve with 1 slice whole-grain bread or roll.

DODGING VITAMIN B12 DEFICIENCY

If you are vegan or you don't eat adequate amounts of animals foods, you and your breastfed baby could be at risk for a deficiency in vitamin B12, which is found naturally only in animal foods. It's especially important for you to take a daily multivitamin with at least 100 percent of the Daily Value for vitamin B12, whether you're breastfeeding or not. Include vitamin B12–fortified foods in your eating plan, too—for example, breakfast cereals, soy and other plant-based beverages, nutrition bars, meat substitutes, and fortified brewer's yeast.

BREASTFEEDING BASICS

Your child is ready to breastfeed just moments after birth. That will be obvious when you see how instinctively he roots for your breast while being held close. It may seem ironic that your milk doesn't fully "come in" until a few days after delivery, but that's because your body knows how much food your child needs, and when. During the initial days after your baby is born, he gets colostrum, or "first milk," from you, which consists of a clear or yellow fluid. Colostrum provides what your child needs just after birth, including antibodies, which are disease-fighting compounds. You won't make much colostrum, but that's OK. Baby's tummy is tiny, and he is getting what he needs for now.

Your breasts will swell and feel warm and tender as your milk production increases. Frequent breastfeeding is important because it stimulates your breasts to produce more milk, which helps build up a steady milk supply. Feed your baby as often as she wants to eat; it's good for your child and alleviates breast discomfort for you, too. You'll know when it's time to nurse by your baby's wide-open eyes and sucking motions.

Breastfeed before fussiness or hunger sets in; otherwise it may be difficult for your baby to calm down and eat. Allow somewhat sleepy babies
to wake up a bit first before feeding.

Breastfeeding a baby is a natural bodily function, but it doesn't always
come naturally to women, and it may be especially trying to those who
are breastfeeding for the first time, or who have had a difficult labor and
delivery, or both. You may have received excellent instructions about
breastfeeding your baby and received wonderful support from the staff
at the hospital, but now that you're home and on your own, you may be
thinking twice about this breastfeeding business. You are not alone; it's
normal for nursing mothers, particularly first-timers, to feel overwhelmed
during the initial weeks after delivery, and possibly for longer.

Giving up on nursing is especially tempting when you're having pain
or discomfort associated with breastfeeding. Try getting some help for
whatever problem you're having before you throw in the towel. Even if
you don't have friends or family who are knowledgeable about breastfeeding, there are plenty of others, including certified lactation consultants,
who are willing to help you learn to nurse your child.

Lactation consultants, who work in hospitals and other settings,
often make house calls and can help you work through the rough spots
you have at any time. Lactation consultants
are knowledgeable about a variety of issues,
including feeding a preterm baby and combin-
ing a return to working outside the home with
breastfeeding. An International Board Certified Lactation Consultant (IBCLC) is a health
care professional, just like a nurse or registered
dietitian nutritionist. IBCLCs are certified by
the International Board of Lactation Consultant Examiners. Visit the International Lacta-
tion Consultant Association's website at www.ilca.org to find a certified
lactation consultant in your area. Your health insurance plan may cover
the services of a lactation consultant.

Sleep deprivation can also prompt thoughts of giving up on breastfeeding. You may take some comfort in knowing that newborns generally do

not sleep through the night for the first few months, regardless of what they eat. Switching to infant formula will not help your baby to sleep for longer stretches. In fact, whether bottle-fed or breastfed, newborns should eat about eight to twelve times a day. They really should not go any longer than four hours without eating during the first three or four weeks, which requires nighttime feedings.

NOTHING BUT THE BREAST

The American Academy of Pediatrics recommends only breast milk for breastfed babies for about the first six months of life. There is no need to give your baby water or any other liquids or solids, although it's fine to start solid foods between four and six months of age, depending on your baby's readiness. The goal is to continue nursing after solid foods are introduced and for at least twelve months. Continue breastfeeding after your baby's first birthday for as long as you and your child desire.

INFANT FORMULA PREPARATION

Always follow the manufacturer's directions for formula preparation. That might seem somewhat obvious, but parents don't always heed the advice. Research has found that one-third of the mothers who were surveyed used warm water directly from the tap to mix infant formula even though the recommendation is to use safe, cold water that has been boiled and cooled. In the same study, nearly half of the mothers heated baby bottles in a microwave oven, a practice that's discouraged because of the risk of burns to a baby's mouth. The American Academy of Pediatrics advises that if you are concerned or uncertain about the safety of tap water, you may use bottled water or bring cold tap water to a rolling boil for 1 minute (no longer), then cool the water to room temperature for no more than 30 minutes before it is used.

The quality of the water used to make infant formula matters. Your house, apartment, or condominium might have pipes made from lead, particularly if the building you live in was constructed prior to 1988.

Lead pipes can leach lead into drinking water. More recent dwellings use copper pipes, but that may not necessarily be safer, as copper pipes can be connected with lead solder that gets into tap water, too. Make sure your water supply is lead-free before you use it for infant formula. See chapter 6 for more on lead.

FOCUS ON FLUORIDE

Fluoride is important to tooth development, particularly before a child's primary teeth start showing through their gums. Although the water supplies in most US cities and towns contain added fluoride—a mineral that can help teeth and nails to grow strong—the levels can be low in certain areas, and your child may need a prescription fluoride supplement. Ask the officials in your town how many parts per million of fluoride are in your drinking water. The American Academy of Pediatrics advises that fluoride supplementation begin at six months and continue through three years of age if the fluoride levels in a child's drinking water are below 0.3 parts per million (ppm). The water from private wells doesn't contain added fluoride, but it may have natural fluoride. If you have a home well, the Environmental Protection Agency recommends having a sample of your water analyzed by a laboratory at least once every three years. Check with the manufacturer about the fluoride content of the bottled water you use to make infant formula. Boiling water does not affect its fluoride level.

IS YOUR BABY EATING ENOUGH?

Babies are great self-regulators—they know when they are full, so they should be allowed to eat as much or as little as they desire. A baby who is satisfied will release the nipple and turn away from the breast. Never force a child to eat, but do encourage your baby to nurse long enough to soften at least one breast during every feeding (start with the other breast for the next feeding). The richer, fattier milk, called hind milk, becomes available later in the feeding.

Nursing newborns should eat eight to twelve times a day during the first month. Your child should have at least six wet diapers every twenty-four hours and three bowel movements a day by the end of the first week of life and should be steadily gaining weight. Ask your pediatrician if you have doubts.

Your child's health care provider will probably want to check your child between three and five days after birth to determine if he or she is gaining an adequate amount of weight. Babies typically experience growth spurts, so be prepared for eating to increase between eight and twelve days old, at about three to four weeks old, and at three months of age. Growth spurts vary thereafter through the first year of life.

> ### Words of Motherly Wisdom
>
> "When I was a new mom, I was concerned that my baby wasn't eating enough because other babies seemed bigger than she was. I was relieved when my pediatrician told me that infants grow at their own pace and that my child was gaining the right amount of weight."
>
> —Peg

IS IT COLIC?

Newborns fuss, and that's to be expected. Fussing is how your baby lets you know that he needs something. However, inconsolable crying jags that occur nearly every day and typically later in the afternoon and early evening, and that last for more than about three hours, are another matter. Your child may have colic.

An estimated 20 percent of babies experience colic, which typically shows up between the second and fourth weeks of life. A child's colicky crying usually ends at around three to four months of age, but it may last until six months. Infants cry to try to soothe themselves, and sometimes it's difficult to break the crying cycle, which is why infants go on and on.

Colic can be caused by several factors, and there's no single explanation for it. Clearly, children with colic are in great discomfort. A colicky child could be sensitive to stimulation or be uncomfortable because of intestinal gas. He or she may make fists and extend or pull up their legs as they pass gas or a bowel movement. Before labeling your child with colic, check with your pediatrician to be sure your child's distress is not due to a medical problem, such as a hernia, or reflux, in which the stomach contents flow backward into the esophagus, causing a burning sensation.

Diet can make a difference in children with colic. Hungry babies may cry incessantly; overfed children may, too. Do not overfeed your baby; it could make her uncomfortable. In general, try to wait at least two to two-and-a-half hours from the start of one feeding to the start of the next one. If bottle feedings take less than twenty minutes, the hole in the nipple could be too large, leading to a bellyache for the baby. Milk protein in infant formula can irritate a baby's intestinal tract. Talk to your pediatrician about a protein hydrolysate formula. If food sensitivity is causing the discomfort, the colic should decrease within a few days of making these changes.

Breastfed children with colic might not tolerate certain foods in their mothers' diets. It's probably a good idea to avoid caffeine when breast-feeding to limit stimulation in your child. Maybe you've heard that nursing mothers should avoid gas-producing foods such as broccoli, onions, and cabbage, and should eliminate milk products and other potentially irritating foods. Although there's not much evidence that this approach alleviates colic in a breastfed baby, if you find that any food is particularly irritating for your child, leave it out of your diet for the time being. If you eliminate entire food groups, you will need to make up for missing nutrients with other nonirritating foods or dietary supplements.

The milk at the end of emptying each breast, called the hind milk, is far richer and is sometimes more soothing. To make sure baby is getting the most hind milk, let him finish nursing on the first breast before offering the second. Offer him the second breast the next time he wants to eat.

Figuring out how best to comfort your colicky child is a matter of trial and error. What works for one baby may not calm another. Swaddle your colicky infant and hold him as much as possible to reassure him, even when he is not crying. Rock him when possible to help him fall asleep. Gently rub your child's back as he lies across your knees, tummy down, but don't allow him to sleep on his stomach, which increases the risk for SIDS. Holding a baby upright can also help to relieve his or her intestinal distress. Put your baby in a car seat and go for a drive. Try an infant swing if your baby is at least three weeks old and can hold his or her head up.

Generally speaking, colicky infants are as likely as those without colic to eat well and gain weight normally. Call your pediatrician or nurse practitioner immediately if your baby's behavior or crying pattern changes suddenly or if your crying child has a fever, forceful vomiting, diarrhea, bloody stools, or anything else out of the ordinary.

REALITY CHECK: GOT COLIC? GET RELIEF

As you work your way through each day with a colicky child, you may take some comfort in knowing that colic does not last forever. But how will you fare while you wait it out? Your child's incessant crying can feel like torture, especially when you're overtired, have other children to care for, or have a job. It would be a miracle if you didn't feel tense, anxious, or angry, or all the above. Parents with colicky children need to know their limits. Ask friends and family members to stay with the baby, even if only for an hour—and get out of the house. You need to remove yourself from the stressful situation to help you maintain a positive attitude and to keep up your strength. Always seek professional help if you're feeling completely overwhelmed and you have thoughts of harming yourself or your baby.

WHEN TO START EXERCISING AFTER GIVING BIRTH

You just had a baby, and it seems as if you're in constant motion as you try to run the household, work in or outside the home, and take care of your baby. You'd like to get back to the gym or some of your usual exercise, and you're wondering when that will be possible.

Take it easy for the first few weeks. While gentle exercise can be energizing, pushing yourself too hard too early after delivery can sap the energy required to care for your new baby. Overdoing physical activity can even be risky, especially if you lost a lot of blood during childbirth, had a cesarean delivery, delivered more than one baby, or were on bed rest for weeks or months before the delivery.

Typically, women get approval for working out at their six-week checkup, but if everything went well during pregnancy and delivery, you may be able to begin walking for exercise within a few weeks after having a child; others will need to wait longer, however. Discuss your situation with your health care provider. Once you get the go-ahead, a gradual return to your prepregnancy level of physical activity is the best strategy.

If you had a cesarean delivery, you know that you've undergone major abdominal surgery. Like all women, you will be encouraged to return to exercise as soon as it is safe to do so, but it will take a bit longer for you. Women who have had cesarean deliveries may be advised to avoid climbing stairs or lifting heavy objects until the wound has healed. Walking only very short distances at first is the best path to recovery. Don't do anything that causes pain or discomfort. There's no point in rushing to exercise. Ask your health care provider what's right for you.

Even if you want to work out, you might be wondering if it's worth spending what little free time you have away from your baby at an aerobics, yoga, or Pilates class. You may prefer to get exercise that allows you to include your baby. Take a walk with the baby in the carrier or the stroller. When the weather is bad, use an exercise DVD, or tune into a cable TV or online exercise program at home, and bounce around the room while your baby watches.

Exercise can help you to lose weight as long as you're eating the right number of calories to shed pounds. A combination of calorie reduction and regular physical activity helps you to drop the pounds while preserving muscle tissue and promoting good health. Keeping the muscle you have, and making more, helps you to burn more calories all day long, because muscle tissue requires more energy to maintain.

You need regular exercise even if weight loss is not your goal. Physical activity is important for women of all ages because it helps to prevent pounds from creeping on as you age, which can help you dodge chronic conditions such as type 2 diabetes. Physical activity also builds and tones muscles, increases stamina and cardiovascular fitness, and enhances mental health.

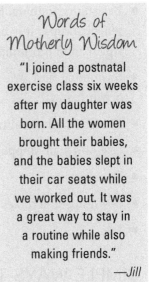

Breastfeeding mothers who exercise intensely should try to feed their babies just before working out for prolonged periods to avoid discomfort and to avoid any potential problems with lactic acid buildup in milk. Working muscles produce lactic acid that gets into breast milk. Lactic acid is not harmful to the baby, but some infants might not like the taste. Try breastfeeding an hour after exercise to improve your baby's acceptance. Drink adequate fluids before, during, and after exercise to stay hydrated. It's unlikely that moderate-intensity exercise will produce enough lactic acid to bother baby.

Words of Motherly Wisdom

"I joined a postnatal exercise class six weeks after my daughter was born. All the women brought their babies, and the babies slept in their car seats while we worked out. It was a great way to stay in a routine while also making friends."

—*Jill*

SQUEEZE IN EXERCISE: SHORT WORKOUTS

It's not always possible to include the suggested minimum of thirty continuous minutes of physical activity when you're busy with baby, but you may find time to get the activity you need every day by dividing it up into ten-minute blocks. Start off with one ten-minute block of activity each day and work your way up to at least three. You can string them together or mix and match different types of exercise. For example, take a brisk thirty-minute walk, or ride a bike for twenty minutes and do resistance training for ten minutes. Following are some activities that fit nicely into one or more ten-minute blocks:

- Walking (a fifteen-minute mile) at the mall, during a coffee break or a lunch break, on a treadmill, or while pushing your child in a stroller

- Slow jogging

- Bicycle riding (at a rate of ten miles per hour)

- Resistance training. Repeat this sequence for ten minutes: ten sit-ups, ten push-ups, ten bicep curls with light to moderate weights, ten squats, and ten jumping jacks

- Swimming and water aerobics (easiest if you have a pool, lake, or ocean handy!)

- Use of an elliptical machine

- Use of a stair-stepping machine

- Dancing

- Low-impact aerobics

- Yoga

SIMPLE WAYS TO BURN CALORIES

It may come as a surprise that many everyday low-level activities are calorie burners that can help you lose some pregnancy pounds, maintain a healthier weight for life, and contribute to overall health and well-being. The following activities burn about 100 calories for a 150-pound person in the amount of time listed. If you weigh more, you'll burn more. If you weigh less, you'll burn less.

Do This	For This Many Minutes
Run up the stairs	6
Walk up the stairs	11
Run in place	11
Kick a soccer ball around	13
Shovel snow	15
Play hopscotch	18
Shoot hoops	20
Mow the lawn	20
Play golf (no cart)	20
Do light yard work	20

Play tag with your children	22
Fly a kite	22
Ride a bike (about ten miles per hour)	22
Toss a Frisbee	29
Carry a small child	29
Wash the car	30
Bowl	30
Throw a ball with your children	30
Explore the zoo while pushing a child in a stroller	35
Sit and play with your toddler	35
Stretch gently	35

Adapted from Ainsworth, B., et al. "Compendium of Physical Activities: An Update of Activity Codes and MET Intensities." *Medicine & Science in Sports and Exercise*, 32(9 Suppl): S498–504, 2000.

WORK IT OUT TOGETHER

Now that you have a baby, your social network will probably get bigger, and that could benefit your fitness efforts. Consider joining a mother-and-baby stroller-walking and fitness group, and find another mom or two to walk with or to swap babysitting with while you work out at home or at the gym.

IDENTIFYING POSTPARTUM DEPRESSION

Like nearly all mothers, you find it challenging to live up to the increased demands on your limited time and fading energy. Do you cry for no real reason? Maybe you lash out at your loved ones even when they are trying to be helpful. Perhaps you're harboring intense feelings of anger and resentment as you get out of bed to feed your infant for the third time that night while your partner, and everyone else in the house, sleeps soundly. You may have more than a case of the "baby blues," which is generally classified as feelings that include worry, unhappiness, and fatigue, and that last for about a week after delivery.

Postpartum depression is a serious medical condition that can develop any time during the first year of your baby's life. It's marked by mood swings, weepiness, an inability to concentrate, and anxiety that hangs on well after the baby is born. The exact causes are unclear, but rapid changes in hormone levels, the physical and emotional stress of giving birth, sleep deprivation, and disappointment about your life now are some of the reasons experts cite for postpartum depression.

Some postpartum moodiness is normal, but problems arise when your feelings interfere with your ability to care for yourself and your child. If you feel anxious, hopeless, or constantly irritable; if you have trouble sleeping even when your baby is asleep; if you feel little connection between you and your newborn; or if you fear harming yourself or your child, you may be suffering from postpartum depression. Women who experienced depression during pregnancy or after a previous pregnancy are particularly prone to the condition.

It's important that you receive treatment, such as talk therapy and support groups, medication, or both, for the way you feel. When a mother is depressed for any reason, she, and every member of her family, particularly infants and young children, are affected. For example, depressed mothers spend less time looking at, talking to, and touching their babies, activities that foster brain development and inspire feelings of trust in the child. Depressed mothers are also less likely to be sensitive to the child's emotional needs. In addition, when you're not feeling well, you may not to eat a healthy diet or exercise as much as you should, which can worsen depression.

LIFE AFTER DELIVERY DAY

During your pregnancy, you may have been motivated more than ever to eat right, exercise, and get the rest you needed. After a child arrives on the scene, life often gets in the way of your best intentions, but it's important to roll with the punches and keep working toward a healthy lifestyle. Now that you have a bigger family, it will serve you and your loved ones well.

You adore your new baby so much that perhaps you're already thinking about having another child. Whether you should do anything differently before the next pregnancy than you did this time depends on your past pregnancy experience and other factors. It is possible to conceive when you're breastfeeding, so use birth control if you don't want to be pregnant just yet. It's never too early for women and their partners to prepare for pregnancy—again!

The next chapter deals with everyday ways to help keep your family healthy. The food choices you make, and the way you handle and prepare foods, influence your well-being when you're pregnant, when you're not, and during breastfeeding. Read on for the latest food safety information.

6

Food Safety and Other Concerns: Before, During, and After Pregnancy

It's always a good idea to be mindful of the safety and the quality of the food you eat, but it's even more meaningful before and during pregnancy and when breastfeeding. You're more prone to getting sick from food during pregnancy because your immune system is weakened and your baby's immune system is underdeveloped, making it harder for both of you to fend off germs and bacteria that can make you ill. Breastfeeding women also need to stay healthy so that they can nourish their child.

You want to protect your child and yourself as much as possible. For the most part, food safety is in your hands. Armed with some basic knowledge, you can ward off exposure to problematic germs, bacteria, and other potentially harmful substances.

PROBLEMATIC BACTERIA AND OTHER SUBSTANCES

Food has all the qualities desired by bacteria and other substances that can make you sick: water, warmth, and nutrients. Since no food is considered completely sterile, it's always best to handle and store food properly. Bacteria, viruses, and parasites can cause food-borne illness (sickness from eating tainted food), but bacteria are most often to blame. The following are some of the most worrisome bacteria (and other substances) for pregnant women.

Listeriosis

Listeriosis is an infection caused by *Listeria monocytogenes* (*Listeria*), a bacterium with the potential for serious consequences for a mother and her unborn child, including miscarriage, stillbirth, preterm labor, and illness or death in newborns. Pregnant women are about twenty times more likely than the general population to get listeriosis. About one-third of all listeriosis cases occur in pregnant women.

Pregnant women with listeriosis may not feel sick right away. Symptoms can take a few days or weeks to appear, and may be mild enough that you don't suspect listeriosis for causing your fever, chills, muscle aches, diarrhea, or upset stomach. If the infection spreads, you may have a headache, stiff neck, confusion, loss of balance, and convulsions. Call your health care provider immediately if you have any symptoms of listeriosis. An infection can be confirmed with a blood test, and you can take antibiotics to treat it. Babies born with listeriosis also receive antibiotics.

As bacteria go, *Listeria* is unusual. Most bacteria grow at temperatures above about forty degrees Fahrenheit, which is the maximum temperature (or should be) of your refrigerator, but *Listeria* can also grow below that temperature, although it reproduces more slowly at lower temperatures.

Listeria is capable of contaminating refrigerated, ready-to-eat deli meats and hot dogs, as well as fruits and vegetables, most notably sprouts, such as alfalfa. Adequate cooking and pasteurization kills *Listeria*. Cover foods well and clean up all refrigerator spills immediately to reduce the risk of spreading bacteria.

Head off listeriosis with these helpful tips:

- Heat hot dogs and luncheon meats, such as ham, turkey, and bologna, to steaming hot, 165°F.

- Avoid soft cheeses such as feta, Brie, Camembert, blue-veined cheese, *queso blanco, queso fresco,* and *queso panela*—unless they're made with pasteurized milk. Check the label to be certain.

- Don't eat refrigerated pâtés or meat spreads or refrigerated smoked seafood, including smoked salmon, trout, whitefish, cod, tuna, and mackerel. These products may be labeled *nova-style, lox, kippered, smoked,* or *jerky.* They are typically offered in the refrigerator section or sold at deli counters of grocery stores and delicatessens. It's fine to have these products if they are part of a properly cooked dish, such as a casserole.

- Avoid raw (unpasteurized) milk or foods that contain unpasteurized milk.

- Always rinse raw produce thoroughly under running tap water before eating.

Toxoplasmosis

Toxoplasmosis is caused by a parasite known as *Toxoplasma gondii (T. gondii).* If you get toxoplasmosis (which means that *T. gondii* is in your bloodstream) when you're pregnant, the parasite can pass through the placenta and harm your unborn child. In babies, toxoplasmosis is capable of causing hearing loss, intellectual disabilities, and blindness. Some children who are born to mothers with toxoplasmosis may not have symptoms at birth but can develop brain or eye problems years later.

Your health care provider may suggest a blood test to check for antibodies to *T. gondii* if you are expecting a child. Generally speaking, if you have been infected with *T. gondii* before becoming pregnant, your unborn child is protected by your immunity. If you are infected during pregnancy, medication is available. You and your baby should be closely monitored during your pregnancy and after your baby is born.

Raw or undercooked meat is a source of *T. gondii.* Other sources are unwashed fruits and vegetables, contaminated water, dust, soil, dirty kitty-litter boxes, and outdoor areas where cat feces are found. *T. gondii* infects just about all cats that spend any time out of the house. Since *T. gondii* doesn't make your cat sick, you probably won't know if your pet harbors the parasite.

You can become exposed to *T. gondii* by an accidental ingestion of contaminated cat feces, which can occur if you touch your unwashed hands to your mouth after you've been gardening, cleaning a litter box, or touching anything that comes in contact with cat feces. Most people infected with *T. gondii* are unaware of it. Some people may feel like they have the flu; they experience swollen glands, fever, headache, muscle pain, or a stiff neck that lasts for a month or more.

You can greatly reduce your risk for toxoplasmosis by:

- Avoiding raw or undercooked meat (see page 189 for safe cooking temperatures) and thoroughly washing raw fruits and vegetables.

- Having your cat's litter box changed daily (the parasite does not become infectious for one to five days after it has been shed in cat feces). Avoid changing the litter box yourself. If that's impossible, wear gloves while changing the kitty litter.

- Wear gloves when gardening or handling sand from a sandbox; cover sandboxes whenever possible to keep cats out.

- Don't get a new cat when you're pregnant.

- Feed your cat commercial dry or canned food, not raw or uncooked meats.

E. Coli Infections

Escherichia coli (*E. coli*) bacteria normally live in the intestines of humans and animals. *E. coli* consists of a diverse group of bacteria. One particular category of *E. coli* bacteria can cause diarrhea, urinary tract infections, respiratory illness, bloodstream infections, and other illnesses. *E. coli* infections are typically caused by *Escherichia coli* O157:H7, the most powerful of hundreds of strains of the bacterium *Escherichia coli*.

Abdominal cramps and bloody diarrhea within two to eight days of eating contaminated food are signs of *E. coli* infection. In most cases, these symptoms last about a week, but a pregnant woman's health may suffer more from the effects of an *E. coli* infection. *E. coli* infections are also serious in young children because they can cause hemolytic uremic syndrome, a condition in which the body's red blood cells are

destroyed and the kidneys can fail. Most healthy people recover from
E. coli infections within ten days. Talk with your health care provider if
you think you have any symptoms of *E. coli* infection.

Undercooked or raw beef tainted with the bacteria is often the source
of *E. coli*. *E. coli* can get into the water supply used for farming, which
is why fresh produce may become infected, too. Here's how to avoid *E.
coli* as much as possible:

- Avoid raw milk and other unpasteurized dairy products and unpasteurized juice, including fresh apple cider.

- Wash your hands thoroughly after using the bathroom, changing diapers, and before preparing or eating food, as well as after contact with
  animals at home, at farms, and petting zoos.

- Cook meats thoroughly. See page 189 for proper cooking temperatures.

- Do not eat raw dough or batter, for cookies, cake, or bread, for example. Flour can be a source of *E. coli*.

- Prevent cross-contamination. See page 189 for more on this topic.

- Avoid swallowing water in swimming pools, lakes, ponds, and streams.

Salmonella Infections

Salmonella infections are caused by a group of bacteria known as
Salmonella. The symptoms of salmonella infection include diarrhea,
fever, and abdominal cramps that begin twelve to seventy-two hours
after exposure to the bacteria. The illness usually lasts from four to
seven days, and most people recover without treatment. However,
some will require hospitalization for severe diarrhea. Pregnant women
may need antibiotics to resolve the infection. A small percentage of
people infected with salmonella develop joint pain, eye irritation, and
painful urination.

Foods contaminated by salmonella usually look and smell normal.
Animal foods, such as beef, poultry, raw milk, and raw eggs, are more
likely to contain salmonella, but all foods, including vegetables, are prone
to contamination. Proper cooking typically kills the bacteria. Pasteurization of milk and treatment of municipal water supplies are highly

effective prevention measures that have been in place for decades to reduce salmonella levels.

Lower the likelihood of salmonella making you sick by taking the following steps:

- Avoid dishes with raw eggs that may not be recognizable as such, including homemade hollandaise sauce, homemade ice cream, Caesar salad dressing, homemade eggnog, mayonnaise, and tiramisu.

- Cook meat to the correct temperature. See page 189 for more information.

- Avoid raw or unpasteurized milk as well as other dairy products made from unpasteurized milk.

- Thoroughly wash raw fruits and vegetables under running water.

- Avoid eating raw cookie dough, cake batter, or other batter containing raw, unpasteurized eggs.

Lead

In the 1970s, the Environmental Protection Agency (EPA) banned the use of lead in gasoline, paint, and many other products. Although lead levels in our environment are on the decline, lead lingers and can cause major health problems.

Lead can accumulate in the body, where it is stored in tissues, blood, and bones. Lead is capable of crossing the placenta and can pass from mother to infant in breast milk. Unborn babies and very young children run the greatest risk of damage when exposed to lead. During pregnancy, exposure to excessive lead can cause miscarriage, low birth weight, preterm delivery, and developmental delays in infants.

Lead-based paint, found mostly in homes built before 1988, and the dust it produces as it deteriorates are major sources of lead exposure. Home repairs such as sanding or scraping paint can create lead dust that's impossible to see, and you can breathe in lead dust without realizing it. Pregnant women, infants, and children should not be in a house with lead paint that's being renovated. If you live in an older home, have it checked by a licensed lead inspector.

Drinking water can pose another lead risk. The EPA estimates that drinking water contaminated with lead can account for 20 percent or more of a person's total exposure to lead. Infants who consume mostly infant formula can receive 40 percent to 60 percent of their exposure if their formula is prepared with lead-contaminated water. Boiling water does not destroy lead.

WHAT'S IN YOUR WATER?

The National Primary Drinking Water Regulations are legally enforceable standards that apply to public water systems. Most water systems test for lead, and many other potential contaminants, as a regular part of water monitoring. These tests provide a system-wide lead level and do not reflect the conditions about the drinking water in your particular home. If you're concerned about contaminants in your water, have it tested by a state-certified laboratory. You can find one in your area by calling the EPA's Safe Drinking Water Hotline at 800-426-4791 or visiting www.epa.gov/safewater/labs.

You may come into contact with lead if you or anyone in your household works in an auto repair shop, a battery-manufacturing plant, or certain types of construction. To minimize your lead exposure, have the people you live with who work at those jobs change their clothes before coming into the house and keep their work shoes outside of the house. Wash their clothes separately from yours.

Pewter and brass containers and utensils may have lead. Don't cook with pewter or brass containers, serve food in them, or use them to store food. Avoid using leaded crystal to serve or store beverages, and stay away from imported lead-glazed ceramic pottery produced in cottage industries.

Lead is bad news, but diet can help to prevent lead from accumulating in your body. Adequate amounts of calcium, iron, and vitamin C help to guard against lead contamination. If you're concerned about your exposure to lead, get your blood tested. Talk to your health care provider about any medicines or vitamins you are taking. Some home remedies and dietary supplements may have lead in them. It is also important to tell your doctor about any unusual cravings you have such as eating dirt or clay, because they may contain lead.

Lead can leach into water from pipes inside the home or pipes that connect homes to the main water supply pipe. Lead found in tap water is usually the result of decaying, old lead-based pipes and fixtures, or from lead solder that connects drinking water pipes. Brass or chrome-plated brass faucets and fixtures with lead solder can contribute significant amounts of lead to the water in your home, especially hot water. Homes built before 1988 are more likely to have lead pipes, fixtures, and solder. Testing is the only way to confirm if lead is present in your home's drinking water. Home water-filtration systems may remove lead from your water, but check to be sure.

Endocrine Disruptors

The endocrine system is a complicated network of hormones and glands, including the thyroid, the pancreas, and the ovaries. The endocrine glands release hormones into the bloodstream that regulate many bodily functions, including energy level, growth and development, and reproduction.

Endocrine disruptors are chemicals that can interfere with the body's endocrine system. Though the evidence is from animal studies, experts say endocrine disruptors can play havoc with the body because they can mimic the estrogen, androgen, and thyroid hormones found naturally in the body, possibly causing overstimulation. Endocrine disruptors can also block the normal function of these natural hormones, and can interfere or block how natural hormones and their receptors are made or controlled.

According to the National Institute of Environmental Health Studies, research shows that endocrine disruptors may pose the greatest risk during pregnancy and early life because that's when organs and the nervous system form. Endocrine disruptors can be natural compounds, such as the phytoestrogens found in certain plant foods, or they can be synthetic substances. The following are some man-made chemicals that can act as endocrine disruptors:

- Bisphenol A (BPA) is a chemical produced to make plastics and resins, and often used in the lining of cans and other containers that store food and beverages, such as water bottles.

- Polychlorinated biphenyls (PCBs) are a category of chemicals that were used to insulate or cool electrical transformers, that were part of hydraulic fluid, and that functioned as lubricants for machinery. PCBs were banned from use by the US government in the 1970s, but because PCBs do not readily break down, they can remain for long periods in the environment, and they can travel. PCBs are found all over the world.

• Dioxin and dioxin-like compounds are by-products of a range of processes, including chlorine bleaching of paper pulp and the manufacturing of some herbicides and pesticides. Like PCBs, dioxins hang around in the environment for years before completely disintegrating.

Endocrine disruptors can be difficult to avoid because they are found in a range of products, such as plastic water bottles, metal food cans, and pesticides. Many endocrine disruptors, including dioxins, are stored in the fat tissue of humans and animals. You can avoid some endocrine disruptors when you eat more of a plant-based diet and choose lean meats and fat-free and low-fat dairy foods most of the time. Reduce your use of canned foods as many cans are lined with a resin that contains BPA. Look for cans and plastic food containers labeled as BPA-free, and choose foods that are in Tetra Pak cartons or glass containers. If a plastic product isn't labeled, keep in mind that plastics marked with recycle codes 3 or 7 may be made with BPA. Don't heat food in the microwave in polycarbonate plastic containers or wash them in the dishwasher. Heat breaks down the plastic and allows BPA to leach into foods and drinks. It's best to heat and store foods and beverages in glass containers. The Food and Drug Administration has banned the use of BPA in plastic baby bottles and sippy cups, and in the coatings of packages of infant formula.

SIMPLE STEPS TO SAFER FOOD

Although troubling bacteria and other substances may lurk in our food, most of the time food is safe to eat, especially when handled properly. Now that you're pregnant, err on the side of caution with these five basic principles of food safety.

Shop Smart

Make sure that all the food you buy is in good condition. Meat, poultry, and dairy foods should be as fresh as possible; check the expiration or sell-by date to be sure. Pick up the cold and frozen foods on your list, such as meat and dairy products, from the grocery store shelves last, just before paying. Go directly home, and put the refrigerated and frozen foods away immediately to preserve freshness. If you won't be returning home for thirty minutes or more after completing your grocery shopping, take a cooler with you to keep foods cold. Consume ready-to-eat, highly perishable foods, such as dairy products, meat, seafood, and produce, as soon as possible after you buy them, or freeze them if you plan to eat them later and not right away.

REALITY CHECK: IS IT OK TO EAT?

You want to minimize food waste, but you don't want to take any chances with your health. Studying the dates on meat, poultry, dairy foods, and eggs can help. Here's what the dates mean:

- The **Sell-By** date informs the store about when to pull the food from its shelves. Buy products with sell-by dates farthest in the future.

- The **Best If Used By (or Before)** date is the time frame for when the food will be at its highest quality and best flavor. This date has nothing to do with safety.

- The **Use-By** date is the last day that the food will be at its peak quality.

When in doubt about a food's safety, throw it out. It's not worth the risk to eat food that may make you sick, especially during pregnancy and when breastfeeding. Go to this website to see how long food is good after you open it: http://www.foodsafety.gov/keep/charts/storagetimes.html.

Keep Hands and Utensils Clean

Before you handle food, always wash your hands thoroughly (for at least twenty seconds) with warm, soapy water. Wash your hands again during food handling and preparation if you have wiped your nose, coughed or sneezed into your hand, used the bathroom, changed a diaper, handled dirty laundry, touched a pet, taken out the garbage, or performed any other activity that could transfer germs to your hands. Encourage proper hand washing by your family and guests by making soap and clean towels or paper towels available at every sink in your home. When it's not possible to use soap and warm water, rely on alcohol-based wipes or gel formulas, which are effective for sanitizing the hands.

GOOD BACTERIA, BAD BACTERIA

An obsession with cleanliness has led to a boom in antimicrobial soaps, hand sanitizers, and kitchen cleansers. Ironically, in our quest to get rid of germs that can make us sick, we encourage their growth. Antimicrobial soaps and other cleansing agents that contain chemical ingredients such as triclosan and triclocarban that help harmful bacteria become resistant to antibiotics. In addition, animal studies suggest that triclosan may alter the way hormones work in the body. The Food and Drug Administration no longer allows the sale of over-the-counter soaps and other products containing triclosan, triclocarban and many other ingredients because there is no proof that these products are safe for long-term daily use and are more effective than plain soap and water. The FDA's ruling does not affect hand "sanitizers" or wipes or antibacterial products used in health care settings, such as hospitals, however. To keep bad bacteria at bay in the kitchen, sanitize countertops with the following homemade cleanser: one teaspoon of liquid chlorine bleach mixed with a quart (32 ounces) of clean water. Wipe countertops and cutting boards with the bleach solution, and leave it for about ten minutes before rinsing for the maximum effect.

Clean your cutting boards, dishes, utensils, and countertops thoroughly with dishwashing soap or a cleaning agent that is safe to use on surfaces that come in contact with food. Replace worn cutting boards (including plastic, nonporous acrylic, and wooden boards), because bacteria can grow in the hard-to-clean grooves and cracks. Use separate cutting boards for produce and meat, and sanitize cutting boards after every time you they come in contact with raw animal protein, such as meat, chicken, and fish.

Always rinse raw fruits and vegetables under cold running water before using them. For thick or rough-skinned vegetables and fruits (such as potatoes, carrots, and cantaloupe), use a small vegetable brush to remove the surface dirt. Cut away the damaged or bruised areas on produce, as germs thrive in these moist places.

Keep Certain Foods Separate

Keep raw animal foods, such as meat, seafood, and eggs, away from ready-to-eat foods, like salad greens and chopped fruit, to avoid getting germs from the uncooked animal foods in those foods that you don't cook. Use a separate plate for cooked food. For example, when you're grilling meats or seafood, do not use the same platter, plate, or bowl for the cooked meat or fish that you used for marinating the raw meat or fish.

Cook Food Properly

When food is heated to the proper temperature, cooking destroys harmful bacteria and other food components that can make you ill. You can't tell whether animal foods are safely cooked simply by looking at them or poking them. Rely on a meat thermometer to determine doneness. Cook (and reheat) foods properly, using these handy guidelines:

Type of Food	Cook to At Least
Whole poultry (chicken or turkey; breasts, thighs, legs, wings)	165°F (74°C)
Fresh beef, veal, lamb steaks, roasts, chops	145°F (63°C)
Ground chicken or turkey	165°F (74°C)
Ground beef, veal, lamb, and pork	160°F (71°C)
Fresh pork and ham*	145°F (63°C)

Seafood (fin fish)	145°F (63°C) Or cook until flesh is opaque and separates easily with a fork.
Shrimp, lobster, and shelled clams	Cook until flesh is pearly and opaque.
In-shell clams, oysters, and mussels	Cook until shells open during cooking.
Scallops	Cook until flesh is milky white or opaque and firm.
Eggs**	Cook until the yolks and whites are firm.
Leftovers, casseroles	165°F (74°C)

*Reheat cooked hams packaged in USDA-inspected plants to 140°F and all others to 165°F.

**Let egg dishes, such as quiche and frittatas, reach 160°F (71°C). Do not eat raw or partially cooked eggs in any form.

If you won't be arriving home within two hours of being served at a restaurant, don't take leftovers or any other food with you. When you order takeout, eat the food immediately or refrigerate it right away. Reheat all leftovers to 165°F (74°C). Bring leftover soups, sauces, and gravies to a boil.

WHEN RAW IS RISKIER

You've been enjoying sushi for years without any health problems. Maybe you always order your favorite sandwich with a generous helping of raw sprouts. Perhaps you adore rare steak. When a pregnancy is in your future or is happening now, it's wise to think twice about typical food choices. Raw or undercooked fish, including sushi and sashimi, are more likely than properly cooked fish to contain parasites and bacteria. Raw shellfish (oysters, clams, mussels) is one of the worst offenders for potentially making you sick, so avoid it at all costs, especially now. The same is true for raw or undercooked meat and eggs, and raw milk and other unpasteurized drinks. Sprouts are healthy food, but they should be cooked. Alfalfa, clover, radish, and other sprouts are highly susceptible to bacterial contamination that cannot be washed off, for the most part.

Keep Food Cold

Most bacteria thrive in temperatures from 40°F (4°C) to 140°F (60°C). Discourage the growth of bacteria that can make you sick by maintaining the temperature in your refrigerator at 40°F (4°C) or below and the freezer at 0°F (–18°C). Use a refrigerator thermometer, and check the temperature periodically. Don't pack the refrigerator or freezer too full with food. Cold air must be able to circulate to keep food safe.

Refrigerate or freeze perishables, prepared food, and leftovers within two hours of eating them or preparing them. It's fine to place warm or hot food in the refrigerator; doing so won't harm the food or your refrigerator. Be sure to divide large amounts of leftovers into shallow containers for quicker cooling in the refrigerator. Discard food that's been left out at room temperature (about 70°F or 21°C) for longer than two hours. When the air temperature hits 90°F or above (32°C), pitch the food after one hour.

At outdoor events, use a cooler to keep cold foods cold. Fill the cooler with food and ice or cold packs. A full cooler maintains its cold temperature longer than one that's only partly filled.

MARINADES, MICROWAVES, AND DEFROSTING

Marinating tenderizes meat, poultry, and seafood, and marinades add flavor. Always marinate foods in the refrigerator—not at room temperature. Never reuse a marinade on cooked foods unless you boil it first.

Microwave ovens tend to heat foods unevenly, leaving some cold spots where bacteria can thrive. Fat, fluid, and sugar heat more quickly, so be careful not to burn yourself. Microwaving vegetables makes produce preparation a snap. When you add some liquid to the microwavable dish and cover it, steam forms to kill bacteria. Ensure that food heats evenly by turning the dish several times and stirring soups and stews periodically.

After defrosting food in the microwave, cook the food right away to prevent bacterial growth. Some areas of the food may become warm and begin to cook during defrosting, allowing bacteria to thrive. Cooking food immediately helps to prevent bacterial growth.

If you don't use the microwave to defrost food, there are two other safe choices. Defrost the food in the refrigerator, or wrapped and in cold water, changing the water every thirty minutes to keep it cold. Don't leave foods out on the counter to defrost at room temperature. Any bacteria present in the food will begin to reproduce.

FISH AND SEAFOOD SAFETY

You're a seafood lover, and that's a good thing. Seafood is an important part of a balanced eating plan. Fish and shellfish pack protein, vitamins, and minerals. Though relatively low in saturated fat, fish and shellfish contain varying amounts of omega-3 fats, which play an important role in your future child's vision and brain development, and in your own health.

The 2015–2020 Dietary Guidelines for Americans recommend that adults eat at least two fish meals (8 ounces) weekly and that pregnant and breastfeeding women include even more: three fish meals (8 to 12 ounces) a week. If you've heard that you should avoid fish during your childbearing years, you may be confused by the recommendations to increase your seafood intake.

There are some fish that women in their childbearing years are advised to avoid. The FDA recommends that pregnant and breastfeeding women avoid swordfish, shark, tilefish (from the Gulf of Mexico), king mackerel, orange roughy, marlin, and bigeye tuna. These larger, long-lived ocean fish have higher levels of methylmercury, which is formed when mercury finds its way into waterways. Bacteria that live in oceans, lakes, and other waterways convert mercury to methylmercury, and fish can absorb the methylmercury from their food supply. Methylmercury accumulates in your body and may possibly harm an unborn child's developing nervous system. Some evidence suggests that the selenium in fish may help counteract potential harm from mercury. However, it's still wise to avoid the types of fish known to have the highest mercury levels.

If you're concerned about the safety of eating fish, chances are you can continue to eat your favorite fish during pregnancy, and maybe more of it. Health organizations around the globe, including the Food and Agriculture Organization and the World Health Organization expert panel, suggest that the benefit of eating fish during pregnancy outweighs the potential risk, and that moms who avoid fish and seafood during pregnancy may be missing out on beneficial nutrients for their babies. Recently released advice from the FDA provides more detailed lists of fish that are safe for pregnant and breastfeeding women. The guidelines include suggestions for fish to eat 2 to 3 times a week, such as salmon, canned tuna, shrimp, and tilapia. See www.FDA.gov/fishadvice for more complete information.

Fish/seafood is an easy-to-prepare, versatile food that is rich in DHA, protein, vitamins, and minerals, and relatively low in saturated fat. See chapter 8 for easy and delicious ways to prepare seafood.

SHOULD YOU GO ORGANIC?

Organic milk, meat, produce, and grains are gaining in popularity. Although you might assume that organic food is probably better for you, it's pricey and it can take a bite out of your food budget. Whether or not you should spend the extra cash on organic food depends on many factors, including understanding the differences between organic and conventionally grown food.

The US Department of Agriculture (USDA) has established an organic certification program. Foods labeled as organic meet specific standards that regulate how the food is grown, handled, and processed. Every product labeled as organic must be USDA certified. Producers who sell less than five thousand dollars a year in organic foods do not have to follow this certification, but they are required to adhere to the USDA's standards for organic foods.

Organic plant foods are produced without using synthetic pesticides, fertilizers made with synthetic ingredients or sewage sludge, bioengineering, or ionizing radiation. A government-approved certifier must inspect the farm to ensure that the standards for organic farming are met. In addition to organic farming, there are USDA standards for organic handling and processing. Organic foods contain no synthetic food additives (or only very small amounts), processing aids (substances used during processing foods but not added directly to foods), or other additives such as artificial sweeteners, colorings, flavorings, or monosodium glutamate (MSG).

Like most conventional farming, organic farming practices are designed to encourage soil and water conservation, reduce pollution, conserve biodiversity, support animal well-being and reduce the incidence of animal illness. Organic farmers use specific natural fertilizers, approved methods to reduce pests that damage crops (including certain pesticides), crop rotation, and mulch to manage weeds. Organic farmers cannot use genetically modified organisms (GMOs) in organic products. They cannot plant GMO crops and their animals cannot eat GMO feed. GMO ingredients are not allowed in packaged organic foods.

Organic foods don't necessarily have more nutrients, but they have lower levels of pesticide residues. Although there is some evidence that foods grown and produced without the use of synthetic fertilizers and pesticides are higher in nutrients, there is probably little difference when you eat a balanced, varied diet. In addition, some organic products may still be high in calories, sugar, and salt. And organic foods, including animal products, are prone to transmitting foodborne bacteria, just like conventional foods. Organically produced meat, milk, eggs, fruit, vegetables, and grains do not provide automatic protection from *E. coli* infections, salmonella poisoning, or other foodborne hazards. Organic foods, including unpasteurized juice and milk, have just as much chance as nonorganic foods of harboring the harmful bacteria that cause these conditions, so handle organic foods with care.

What's in a Label?

If a food bears the USDA Organic label, it means it's produced and processed according to the USDA standards. The seal is voluntary, but many organic producers use it.

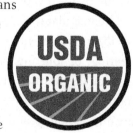

Foods that are completely organic, including produce, eggs, and other single-ingredient foods, can say they are "100% organic" and use the USDA seal. A product that contains 95 percent or more organic ingredients can say it's "organic" and may also display the seal. Foods that contain a minimum of 70 percent but less than 95 percent organic ingredients will read "made with organic ingredients" but cannot display the USDA seal.

PESTICIDES IN PERSPECTIVE

Organic produce is raised without most synthetic fertilizers or synthetic pesticides. In comparison, many different types of man-made pesticides—chemicals that defend crops from pests that would ruin them or reduce their yield—are used on conventional produce in the United States and on imported produce and grains. According to the FDA, the greatest potential for pesticide exposure comes from conventional fruits and vegetables. However, while these foods have higher synthetic pesticide levels than others, the amount does not violate the levels that the FDA considers safe. Depending on the country of origin, imported conventionally grown produce may have more pesticides than produce grown in the United States.

It's hard to say whether harm is caused by the synthetic pesticides and other contaminants in conventional foods, because there is little data available on the long-term safety. Nevertheless, when you are of childbearing age, pregnant, or breastfeeding, it never hurts to avoid as many synthetic chemicals as possible. Pesticides and other chemicals in food and in the environment may be detrimental, especially during vulnerable periods of life, including fetal development and early childhood.

Buying organic produce can minimize, but not completely eliminate, pesticide residues. This fact might come as a surprise to people who are currently spending the extra money for organic foods. Small amounts of pesticide residues are unavoidable even on many organic fruits and

> *Words of Motherly Wisdom*
>
> "I'd like to include more organic foods, but they cost more than regular options. That's why I've decided to buy the organic versions of the four or five foods I eat most often."
>
> —*Peg*

vegetables, because wind and water spread pesticides that have been used on other crops. Furthermore, some pesticides persist in the soil for years and may be absorbed by plants even after the land has been certified organic. Pesticide residues are uncommon in milk, beef, poultry, and eggs.

REDUCE THE RISK

On balance, experts advocate eating adequate amounts of fruits and vegetables, no matter how they are grown. Washing and rinsing fresh produce may lower the level of some pesticides, but it won't completely eliminate them. Peeling also reduces the pesticide level, but valuable nutrients often go down the drain with the peel. To reduce your overall risk, eat a variety of foods; wash produce thoroughly; and consider organic options for the produce you eat often.

ORGANIC MILK, MEAT, AND SEAFOOD

Organic milk is from cows that have been fed an organic diet for at least the past year or during their entire lives, and they have also not been given growth hormones or antibiotics. "Hormone-free milk" does not mean the milk is also organic. There is no such thing as hormone-free milk. That's because milk, even the organic variety, contains, at the very least, low levels of bovine somatotropin (BST), also called bovine growth hormone (BGH), which is produced naturally by cows. Recombinant BST (rBST) is a bioengineered version of natural BST that may be given to cows to boost milk production. Milk from cows given rBST is safe, according to the FDA. The use of rBST is not an issue with certified organic milk, because the USDA standards for organic food state that organic milk cannot come from cows treated with rBST.

Certified organic livestock are managed without antibiotics and added growth hormones. (If antibiotics are given to treat an infection, the animal can no longer be considered organic.) The animals eat 100 percent certified organic feed or grass that's been grown without toxic pesticides or fertilizers, and cannot be genetically engineered. Although "free-range" animals are allowed year-round access to the outdoors, they are not automatically organic; similarly, "naturally raised" provides no guarantee that the meat or poultry from those animals is organic. Wild seafood cannot be labeled as organic. According to the USDA, the certification standards for using the organic label on aquaculture, also known as fish farming or shellfish farming, is under review by the agency.

There's no conclusive scientific evidence that organic milk, meat, and chicken are better for you. It's up to you to choose what types of animal foods to eat.

THE DISH ON FOOD ADDITIVES

When you're unfamiliar with the lingo, studying the ingredients on food labels is like trying to decipher another language with words like *niacinamide, pyridoxine hydrochloride, ferrous gluconate,* and *ascorbic acid* staring back at you. Even though the names are difficult to decode, most food additives are considered safe, including the ones mentioned above, which are the technical terms for common vitamins and minerals in foods and dietary supplements.

There are several reasons for adding certain substances to food. Some additives, like vitamin C (ascorbic acid), promote freshness and boost nutrition; others, like sugar and salt, enhance taste and appearance; still others replace nutrients lost in processing. For example, B vitamins that were stripped away during the making of refined grains, such as white bread, are added back, resulting in an *enriched* product. *Fortified* foods contain nutrients that were not present naturally. Most milk is fortified with vitamins A and D. Iron and folic acid are often added to breads, cereal, and other grains to enhance their nutritional profile.

Some food additives have pitfalls. Sulfites, which may be found in foods such as dehydrated potatoes, dried fruit, some fermented foods, and commercial bread products, may trigger allergies in some people with asthma. Sodium nitrate and sodium nitrite, which provide hot dogs and other cured meats with their pink hue and protect them from germ growth, are potential carcinogens.

If you want to limit food additives, eat a diet rich in fresh and min-imally processed foods. Following that advice will also curb your con-sumption of added sodium and added sugar, which are common food additives. Foods labeled "preservative-free" contain fewer food additives.

BETTER SAFE THAN SORRY

While it's necessary to think about bacteria and other contaminants in food and water, it can be scary. Try not to be alarmed. Despite the possibilities for problems, overall our food supply is quite safe. You can't eliminate all risk, but you can feel more confident knowing how to help yourself and your family stay healthy to the best of your ability.

7

Common Concerns and Special Situations

M any women experience only minor discomforts during pregnancy, while others have more than their fair share of problems. In all likelihood, you will have little to contend with when you're expecting or trying to conceive. Just in case, this chapter delves into some of the most common issues concerning pregnancy and ways to manage them.

AGE

You can't change how old you are. However, based on your particular age, it might be even more important to eat a nutritious diet and live a healthy lifestyle.

Teen Moms

Women under age twenty who are expecting a child have become pregnant before their own bodies have had a chance to fully mature. Adolescents tend to choose low-nutrient foods, preferring soft drinks to milk, french fries to baked potatoes, and fast food instead of more nutritious, homemade fare. Young people also tend to skip meals more often than older people do.

Pregnant teens may not meet their own nutrient needs, particularly for iron, folic acid, and calcium, never mind the increased needs of pregnancy. As a result, a teen mother-to-be and her growing baby may compete for nutrients, shortchanging both in terms of health and development.

MORE CALCIUM, BETTER BONES

Adolescence is when teens accumulate much of the bone mass they will have for life. According to the Institute of Medicine, the group of experts that determines suggested nutrient intakes for people in the United States, pregnant women, including teens, don't require additional calcium because their bodies become more efficient in absorbing calcium during pregnancy. However, teenagers need more calcium than women between the ages of twenty and fifty to begin with: 1,300 milligrams a day, or about the equivalent of four servings of dairy foods as part of a balanced eating plan. A pregnant teen is building up her bone mass at the same time as her baby is building his or her bones. Adequate calcium intake helps both mother and child to lay the foundation for a stronger skeleton.

Teens may tend to enter pregnancy at an unhealthy weight (under- or overweight) more often than their older counterparts, and they are less likely to gain the recommended number of pounds. Adolescent mothers are more prone to preterm delivery (before thirty-seven weeks), iron-deficiency anemia, and elevated blood pressure.

Despite the added challenges, it is possible to have a healthy pregnancy while nourishing a teenage body. These strategies can help:

- Seek regular prenatal care as soon as possible after you find out you're pregnant.

- Take a prescription prenatal vitamin and mineral pill every day. You may need extra dietary supplements, such as calcium, iron, and docosahexaenoic acid (DHA), a healthy fat for baby's brain development.

- Read chapter 3 to help you plan the healthiest diet possible. If you need help, consult an RDN for an eating plan that's tailored to meet your needs. Get a free referral to a dietitian in your area by going to www.eatright.org.

- Check out the government's Special Supplement Program for Women, Infants, and Children, better known as WIC. The WIC program serves low-income pregnant and breastfeeding women and their children up to age five. It provides vouchers for food that are redeemable at grocery stores, nutrition education, and referrals to health services and other organizations—all free of charge. Visit www.fns.usda.gov/wic/women-infants-and-children-wic for the location of an office in your area.

- Eat on a regular basis throughout the day. Have at least three balanced meals. In each snack, try to include foods from at least two of the five food groups, and at each meal try to include foods from at least three food groups.

- Avoid too much caffeine, and all alcohol. See chapter 2 for more information on how much caffeine is safe during pregnancy and breastfeeding.

- Stop smoking cigarettes, hookah, and e-cigarettes.

- Speak with your doctor or pharmacist about any medications and herbal supplements you take to determine their safety during pregnancy. Do not use recreational drugs, illegal or not.

FROM THE RECIPE FILE

Macaroni and Cheese with Butternut Squash (page 260) is a classic favorite with more vegetables than usual. It's packed with calcium and protein, too.

Older Moms

You might have had your last child several years ago and now find yourself pregnant again at age thirty-five, forty, or forty-four. Maybe you're trying for your first baby later in life than you expected. You're not alone. More women than ever are having their first child after their thirty-fifth birthday.

If you already have a family, you may think you know what to expect from pregnancy and childbirth. However, each pregnancy is unique, and a pregnancy after thirty-five or forty may be harder on your body than previous pregnancies. Being an older mom does not mean you will experience complications, but the passage of time means that you're more likely to be managing pregnancy in addition to a health condition, such as type 2 diabetes, high blood pressure, or being overweight. Paying attention to your dietary and lifestyle needs is more important than ever now.

If this is your first pregnancy and you're older than thirty-five, it's a good idea for you to seek preconception care to manage any health problems you might have had before conception. Other than that, the lifestyle advice for healthy older mothers is similar to the suggestions for women in their twenties and early thirties. That's also true if you're having twins, which is more likely over the age of thirty-five.

TWINS (AND MORE) PREGNANCIES

Though still relatively low, the rate of twin births has been rising steadily, and it reached a new national high in 2014. Experts say that assisted reproductive techniques (ART) such as in vitro fertilization are probably the reason for the increase. In addition, older women more often naturally conceive more than one child at a time. You may have more trouble getting pregnant after age thirty-five, but when you do, you're more likely to have twins!

When you're having twins or more, your pregnancy probably won't go to forty weeks. Preterm birth (before thirty-seven weeks) is more common with more than one baby, and your newborns may weigh less at delivery than if you were having just one child. There's a greater chance that you'll develop high blood pressure and gestational diabetes. Expect to see your health care provider more often than if you were pregnant with only one child.

Consult chapter 4 for advice about how much weight to gain with a twin pregnancy. If you began pregnancy with a body mass index in the healthy range, you may be advised to gain between thirty-seven and fifty-four pounds, which is twelve to nineteen more pounds than if you were having just one baby. To put on that many pregnancy pounds, you will need to eat at least 500 additional calories every day, starting in the first trimester. You will also need 50 additional grams of protein daily, starting in the first trimester, too. Speak to your health care provider about how many pounds you should gain.

As for other nutrients, there isn't much scientific evidence about what to eat when having twins, the most common type of multiple pregnancy, and even less for triplets and more. Most diet advice for twin pregnancies is taken from the information we have about women pregnant with one child. It seems sensible to assume that nutrient needs would double in twin pregnancies, but there's no research to prove that's true. However, it's reasonable to think that twin pregnancies require higher levels of nutrients. Some experts recommend more calcium, magnesium, zinc, iron, vitamin C, vitamin E, and DHA. An increased intake of healthy foods and a prescription prenatal supplement will likely satisfy your nutrient needs. You'll probably need to take single dietary supplements for extra vitamin D, calcium, and DHA. Don't go it alone when planning what to eat if you're having more than one child at a time. Consult with a registered dietitian nutritionist (RDN) who specializes in pregnancy about a balanced eating plan.

CONSTIPATION

Constipation is generally defined as moving your bowels three or fewer times a week or having stool that is difficult to pass. When you have constipation, your stools are usually hard, dry, and small in size.

Constipation can set in as early as the first trimester. The pregnancy hormone progesterone may be partly to blame, because it slows the movement of food through your digestive tract. As pregnancy progresses, your expanding uterus puts pressure on your intestines, which also contributes to constipation. High levels of iron in prenatal pills and other dietary supplements can cause constipation, too.

Constipation is common following childbirth and surgery. Labor and delivery are hard on the muscles that are used to pass stool. Your bowels may also be sluggish at first because of medication you received during labor.

The sooner your intestinal tract is in top working order, the better. Here's how to curb constipation:

- **Focus on fiber.** Fiber-rich foods, such as fruits, vegetables, legumes, and whole grains, bulk up stools, making them easier to pass. Aim for at least 28 grams of fiber a day. See chapter 2 for more on fiber sources. Increase your fiber intake slowly to avoid gas and bloating.

- **Drink up.** Liquid adds fluid to the colon, promoting bulkier and softer stools. Pregnant women need at least ten 8-ounce glasses of fluid daily, and nursing women need thirteen. If you're not breastfeeding, aim for nine glasses of fluid. Drinking hot water with lemon or hot tea can help to relax your intestinal tract and add fluid to help promote movement.

- **Walk it off.** Physical activity increases the flow of blood to the intestinal tract, which can help prevent constipation.

> *Words of*
> *Motherly Wisdom*
> "I found [that] including a high-fiber cereal every day, avoiding too much cheese, and munching on dried fruit and nuts worked to relieve my constipation."
> —*Dina*

FROM THE RECIPE FILE

The Go Green Smoothie Bowl (page 231) is a delicious way to curb constipation. One serving supplies 18 grams of fiber as well as fluid from fruit.

HEMORRHOIDS

Constipation is bad enough, but if you have to strain to move your bowels, you may acquire hemorrhoids, which are swollen veins in the rectal area that can become itchy or painful and might bleed. To make matters worse, pregnancy hormones enable the walls of your veins to relax and swell more easily. Pressure on your intestinal tract from a growing baby and sitting or standing for long periods can bring on hemorrhoids, too. Pushing during labor may also cause hemorrhoids.

If you've had hemorrhoids before, you're more likely to develop them during pregnancy. Having hemorrhoids during one pregnancy increases the risk of a flare-up in future pregnancies. Thankfully, hemorrhoids are manageable. Following the advice for avoiding constipation is a good place to start—before, during, and after pregnancy. When you're expecting, stick to the weight-gain guidelines that are right for you, as extra weight makes hemorrhoids more likely to occur.

Ask your health care professional how to manage the discomfort of hemorrhoids. Always check with your provider before using medication to treat hemorrhoids.

HEARTBURN

In spite of the name, heartburn has nothing to do with your heart. *Acid indigestion* is a better name for this sour, burning sensation in the upper abdomen, the chest, or the throat.

Stomach acid is at the root of heartburn. When compounds in the stomach used for digestion stay where they belong, they pose no problem. Heartburn occurs when stomach acid splashes into the esophagus, the tube that carries food from your mouth to your stomach. This backwash occurs because the lower esophageal sphincter, a muscular valve that separates the esophagus and the stomach, relaxes too often. When the sphincter doesn't close often enough, it allows the stomach acid to move upward into the esophagus, causing symptoms of heartburn and, in severe cases, damage to the lining of the esophagus.

Pregnancy's changing hormone levels can be one cause of heartburn. Pregnant women are susceptible to heartburn at any time, but it's also common in the third trimester, when the baby is big enough to crowd your stomach and push stomach contents into the esophagus.

WHEN HEARTBURN HANGS ON

Frequent bouts of heartburn after delivery day has come and gone may be a sign of something more serious than stomach discomfort. If you have heartburn more than two times a week, you could have gastro-esophageal reflux disease (GERD). Treating GERD is important to protect your esophageal lining from damage that could eventually give rise to cancer. Managing GERD may be as simple as changing your diet or taking prescription or over-the-counter medications. Let your health care provider know if you are breastfeeding so that the appropriate medication can be prescribed, if necessary.

Try these techniques to reduce reflux during pregnancy:

- Eat smaller meals throughout the day instead of larger ones, especially at dinner.

- Eat slowly and chew your food completely for better digestion.

- Avoid foods that irritate your condition, which may include spicy foods, tomatoes, fried foods and other greasy fare, chocolate, peppermint, carbonated beverages, and caffeine.

- Drink fluids between meals, not with them. Too many fluids with food can crowd your stomach and encourage reflux.

- Sit up after eating. Prop your head up in bed by six inches to prevent stomach acids from reaching chest level at night. Wait two to three hours after eating before going to bed.

- Chew gum. Chewing stimulates the swallowing of saliva, which buffers acid in the esophagus.

If these measures fail, consult your health care provider about medications to ease acid indigestion. Don't take any medication to treat your heartburn without checking first with your health care provider.

MORNING SICKNESS

Women who suffer from morning sickness will tell you that the nausea and vomiting associated with pregnancy can strike at any time of the day and at any location: in public, driving in the car, and even at work!

Experts are unsure about the cause of the queasiness that's typically one of the first signs of pregnancy, but shifts in hormone levels are probably to blame. A heightened sense of smell caused by hormonal surges can interfere with your attempts to feel better because offensive odors can easily trigger a wave of nausea or a bout of vomiting that wrecks your appetite and saps your energy.

Morning sickness seems to run the gamut: some women are queasy for a few weeks in the first trimester, while others are sick on a daily basis until they deliver. For the most part, morning sickness ends early in the second trimester. When you can't keep a bite of food or even just a few sips of water down, you are likely to wonder if morning sickness is hurting the baby. In general, morning sickness is not harmful to your child unless it persists to the point where you are losing a lot of weight and becoming very dehydrated. Dehydration and weight loss are common in the condition called *hyperemesis gravidarum,* which affects tens of thousands of women every year. Women with hyperemesis gravidarum require medical supervision to ensure the body's proper balance and to monitor their weight and conditions that jeopardize their health.

How do you know if your morning sickness is a cause for concern rather than a passing annoyance? According to the National Institutes of Health, the following are warning signals:

- A loss of two or more pounds in a week

- Severe vomiting that won't stop

- Vomiting blood or material that resembles coffee grounds (call your health care provider immediately if this occurs)

If you're worried that your next pregnancy will be plagued by morning sickness as severely as this one is, try not to be concerned right now. Each pregnancy is unique, and morning sickness with one baby does not mean it will happen again in the future. When morning sickness feels intolerable, try to keep in mind that it always disappears when your pregnancy ends!

The following tips can help you to better manage your morning sickness:

- Don't overdo it. Get plenty of sleep, and relax whenever possible. Stress exacerbates the effects of morning sickness, which includes fatigue.

- Avoid rushing. Allow enough time to get out of bed in the morning and to get ready for the day. Some women leave bland-tasting crackers at their bedside to munch on before they get up.

- Don't let yourself get too hungry. Dips in blood glucose levels can make matters worse. Eat small meals throughout the day, and avoid fatty foods and others that aggravate your stomach.

- Eat what appeals to you, even if it may not be the healthiest of options, as long as it's considered safe during pregnancy. Just remember to return to your MyPlate eating plan as soon as you are able.

- Eat cold or room-temperature foods. Strong smells can trigger nausea, and cold foods are less aromatic than warmer ones.

- Focus on carbohydrates. Plain baked potatoes, toast, rice, and pasta may be easy on the stomach, and they're comforting, too. Choose whole-food and whole-grain varieties as much as possible.

- Take your prenatal vitamins at night, just before going to sleep, or with food, to reduce stomach irritation. Check with your health care provider about switching from your prenatal vitamin to another type of multivitamin (such as a liquid or chewable form) until your morning sickness passes.

- Consider acupressure wristbands, which are often employed to prevent seasick-

> ### Words of Motherly Wisdom
> "I couldn't be anywhere near meat or chicken when it was cooking. The smell of it was overwhelming and would make me sick."
> —*Diane*

ness. Look for them at pharmacies, marine specialty shops, and in health-food stores.

- Try acupuncture to relieve your distress. Look for an acupuncturist who is trained to work with pregnant women.

- Target your triggers. Offensive smells can set you off, limiting your appetite and the ability to keep food down. Reduce your exposure to odors you find unpleasant by keeping rooms well ventilated and avoiding secondhand smoke.

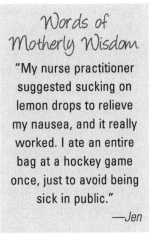

Words of Motherly Wisdom

"My nurse practitioner suggested sucking on lemon drops to relieve my nausea, and it really worked. I ate an entire bag at a hockey game once, just to avoid being sick in public."

—Jen

- Sip ginger tea or flat ginger beer (a nonalcoholic drink). Ginger ale may not contain any real ginger, but it may also help. Peppermint tea is also soothing and is considered safe during pregnancy.

- Nibble on frozen fruit-juice pops for the fluid and the sugar, which provides calories and helps you maintain your energy.

- High doses of vitamin B6—100 milligrams (mg) a day or less—may help to alleviate pregnancy-induced nausea. However, do not take large doses of vitamin B6 or any other vitamin, dietary supplement, or medication without talking to your health care provider first.

FROM THE RECIPE FILE

Make a big batch of Ginger Tea (page 223) to help calm your queasy stomach.

GESTATIONAL DIABETES

Gestational diabetes mellitus (GDM), often called gestational diabetes, is a type of diabetes that occurs in some pregnant woman who did not have diabetes before they became pregnant. In GDM, the glucose (sugar) levels in your bloodstream are too high, which is called *hyperglycemia*.

Hyperglycemia happens because your body is unable to make and use all of the insulin it needs, a condition called *insulin resistance*. Glucose is the source of energy for every cell in your body and your baby's body. Insulin helps glucose to enter your cells, where it is converted to energy. When insulin doesn't function properly, glucose builds up in the blood.

Although glucose is beneficial because it provides energy, too much glucose is not beneficial for you or your baby. When your blood glucose is elevated, your pancreas, the organ that makes insulin, works overtime to make more insulin to compensate for the insulin resistance that occurs during pregnancy. When the pancreas isn't able to make enough insulin to compensate for the insulin resistance, gestational diabetes results. The extra glucose baby receives from you causes his pancreas to also work harder to get rid of the high levels of glucose that enter his bloodstream. Since your baby is getting additional calories as glucose from your blood on a steady basis, he will likely grow large enough to have difficulty being born. Larger infants are prone to shoulder damage during delivery because it's harder for them to get through the birth canal. A cesarean delivery may be required because of the baby's size. Children born to mothers with poorly controlled GDM may have elevated blood glucose levels for hours or days afterward that may require treatment to reduce. They are at greater risk for breathing problems, more likely to become overweight in childhood, and more likely to have diabetes as adults. In addition, mothers with GDM may experience high blood pressure during pregnancy.

The Centers for Disease Control and Prevention estimates that GDM could affect more than 9 percent of all pregnancies in the United States. Experts aren't exactly sure why GDM occurs, but there are definite risk factors, including the following:

- Being over age twenty-five

- Having prediabetes or having a family member who has type 2 diabetes

- Having GDM in a previous pregnancy

- A body mass index (BMI) of 30 or higher

- Being black, Hispanic, American Indian, or Asian

Diagnosing GDM

Your health care provider should test your blood for GDM between twenty-four and twenty-eight weeks of pregnancy. To determine whether you have GDM, you will drink a sugary beverage and receive a blood test to measure your blood glucose level. If your fasting blood glucose concentration is higher than normal, you will have another test to confirm the condition.

Treating GDM

If your GDM test is positive, you should take steps as soon as possible to lower your blood glucose level and keep it within a normal range. GDM is often controlled with diet and regular physical activity. Exercise naturally lowers blood glucose because working muscles use glucose for fuel.

You might also be asked to monitor your blood glucose concentration several times a day, and there's a possibility that you will need insulin injections to normalize blood glucose levels. Ask your health care provider for a referral to an RDN who can help you with a meal plan that's right for you. It takes some work to manage GDM, but it's well worth the time and effort to ensure your and your baby's good health.

After the Baby Arrives

Gestational diabetes disappears once you've delivered your baby. However, having GDM during one pregnancy puts you at greater risk for the condition in future pregnancies. Some women with GDM develop type 2 diabetes after the baby is born. If you have GDM, you need a blood test six to twelve weeks after delivery to see whether your blood glucose is elevated. If your fasting blood glucose level is within the normal range (100 or less) at six to twelve weeks after your baby is born, get your blood glucose tested at least every three years from then on. It's easy for blood glucose levels to creep up with time in women (and in men, too). Throughout life, aim for a fasting blood glucose level of 100 or less to avoid the harmful effects of prediabetes and type 2 diabetes. You can manage blood glucose concentrations by achieving and maintaining a healthy weight and getting regular exercise.

PRETERM BIRTH

Preterm birth—giving birth before thirty-seven weeks—is a common problem in the United States. About one in ten babies is born too early, also called premature birth.

It's important that pregnancy lasts as close to forty weeks as possible because growth and development continue well into the final weeks and months. The earlier a baby is born, the greater the chances for health problems. For instance, babies born at thirty-five weeks are more likely to be low birth weight (less than five pounds eight ounces); have breathing problems because of underdeveloped lungs; and experience jaundice. Jaundice is the buildup of bilirubin in the baby's blood because his liver isn't developed enough to break it down.

Preterm delivery can happen to any woman, but some women are more prone to it than others. Women expecting twins or more babies, those who have had a premature baby in the past, and those who have problems with their uterus or cervix run a greater risk for preterm birth. Certain health conditions—including diabetes, high blood pressure, or being overweight or underweight, among others—influence the risk of preterm birth. Certain lifestyle habits, such as smoking cigarettes or using alcohol and recreational drugs, also increase the likelihood of having a baby born too early.

You may have one or more risk factors for preterm birth, but that does not necessarily mean that your baby will be born before his due date. However, you should take the best possible care of yourself and discuss with your doctor all the ways you can prevent delivering early.

BLOOD PRESSURE DISORDERS

Some women enter pregnancy with high blood pressure, called chronic hypertension, while others develop high blood pressure for the first time when they are expecting, a condition known as gestational hypertension or pregnancy-induced hypertension (PIH). Gestational hypertension begins after twenty weeks of pregnancy. Gestational hypertension may be relatively mild, but it can also be severe and troublesome.

Blood pressure is the force of the blood pushing against the walls of your arteries, which are the blood vessels that transport oxygen-rich blood to every part of the body, including to your unborn child. High blood pressure during pregnancy can cause growth problems for the baby as well as preterm birth.

Your health care provider will measure your blood pressure at every visit during your pregnancy. Blood pressure readings consist of two numbers. The first, or top, number registers systolic pressure, the pressure in the arteries when your heart contracts. The second, or bottom, reading represents diastolic pressure, the pressure in the arteries when the heart relaxes between contractions. Normal blood pressure is considered to be lower than 120 over 80.

If your readings are consistently elevated at your regular prenatal visits, your health care provider may suggest that you have your blood pressure taken more often. A diagnosis of hypertension prior to the twentieth week of pregnancy probably means that you have chronic hypertension and that your blood pressure won't revert to normal once you deliver.

Gestational hypertension doesn't usually harm the mother or baby, and it disappears after delivery. However, about 15 to 25 percent of women with gestational hypertension develop preeclampsia. Preeclampsia occurs when you have a combination of high blood pressure and an abnormal amount of protein in your blood, known as proteinuria. As preeclampsia worsens, pregnant women develop abnormal kidney or liver function, vision changes, and severe headache, among other symptoms.

An estimated 3 to 5 percent of women in the United States develop preeclampsia. Preeclampsia usually shows up after twenty weeks of pregnancy, but it can also happen after you have the baby. Rapid and extreme weight gain (e.g., more than two pounds a week) can signal preeclampsia. It's important to deal with preeclampsia immediately, because it can cause preterm delivery, serious illness, and maternal and fetal death. Left untreated, preeclampsia can progress swiftly to eclampsia. Eclampsia can trigger seizures that cause pregnant women to lose consciousness, fall, and twitch uncontrollably. If left untreated, it may lead to the death of the mother, the baby, or both.

You're more likely to develop preeclampsia if you:

- Are pregnant for the first time
- Had high blood pressure, kidney disease, or both before becoming pregnant
- Are over age forty
- Are pregnant with more than one child
- Have already had a pregnancy affected by preeclampsia
- Have a family history of the condition
- Have diabetes or an immune disorder
- Have a history of drug or alcohol abuse or you smoke cigarettes
- Are obese
- Have a pregnancy that is the result of egg donation, donor insemination, or in vitro fertilization

The good news is that uncomplicated preeclampsia usually disappears within six weeks of giving birth. The not-so-good news is that once you've had preeclampsia, you are more likely to develop high blood pressure and heart disease later in life.

Managing your health to the best of your ability, eating a balanced diet, gaining the recommended number of pounds, and exercising regularly (if your doctor approves) are all ways to reduce the risk of PIH. The role of food and dietary supplements in preventing high blood pressure disorders during pregnancy is not particularly promising, with one possible exception. A review of thirteen studies concluded that taking at least 1,000 milligrams of calcium daily as supplements reduced blood pressure and risk of preeclampsia. It's important to note that taking supplemental calcium may only work to reduce high blood pressure disorders in women whose calcium intakes are very low. However, calcium has been identified by the 2015 Dietary Guidelines for Americans as a nutrient of public health concern, which means that many women are deficient in this nutrient before pregnancy.

SURVIVING BED REST

Health care providers sometimes prescribe bed rest for preterm labor, vaginal bleeding, problems with the placenta, an incompetent cervix (when the cervix is likely to dilate before your due date), and indications that the baby isn't growing properly. Bed rest increases blood flow to the placenta and may increase a baby's birth weight. While bed rest isn't a proven remedy for preventing pregnancy complications or preterm birth, it's still recommended by some practitioners, although less often than in the past.

Bed rest varies. Some women are confined to rest only while they are at home. Others must stay in bed or on the couch all the time, getting up only to use the bathroom. Still other pregnant women are hospitalized to allow virtually no movement.

You may sometimes dream of just sitting and doing nothing, but when inactivity lasts for weeks or months, it gets old fast. Immobility weakens your muscles and reduces the strength of your heart and lungs. Inactivity curbs your appetite, and bed rest may encourage insufficient weight gain and nutrient intake.

REALITY CHECK:
BED REST CAN PRODUCE STRESS

When you have other children or family responsibilities to fulfill, bed rest is a burden and wears on you quickly. Bed rest can be a financial yoke as well, because you are missing out on earning an income and you might also need to hire someone to do the jobs you typically do, such as housecleaning and yard work. You might be able to work from bed. If not, at least you can use the Internet to connect with others in the same situation. Check out groups such as Sidelines High Risk Pregnancy Support (www.sidelines.org) and Mamas on Bedrest & Beyond (www.mamasonbedrest.com).

Ask your health care provider about getting physical therapy to stay as strong as possible while you're on bed rest. Though you're not particularly hungry, it's still important to stick with your pregnancy eating plan as much as possible; eat six or eight small meals a day instead of larger meals that may be more difficult to consume.

DEALING WITH SWELLING

Swelling, or edema, is a normal, common part of pregnancy. It's due to an increase in the production of blood and other body fluids to meet the needs of your growing baby. You may have edema in your hands, face, legs, ankles, and feet. Pressure on your vena cava (the large vein on the right side of the body that is responsible for returning blood to your heart from your lower extremities) and on your pelvic veins make you prone to accumulating fluid in your legs, ankles, and feet.

You'll probably start experiencing edema when you reach your fifth month or so, although swelling can start at any point in your pregnancy. You may notice that your puffiness peaks at the end of the day. A sudden change in fluid balance is a different matter; this may signal preeclampsia, which could endanger you and your baby.

Call your health care provider immediately if you experience sudden swelling. If your blood pressure and your urine are normal, there is probably nothing to be concerned about.

Take the following steps to help diminish normal swelling:

- Avoid sitting or standing for long periods. These activities allow fluid to accumulate in your lower extremities.

- When you sit, elevate your feet.

- Engage in walking or swimming to move fluid out of the affected areas as much as possible. Doing water aerobics is helpful in reducing leg edema in pregnant women. Ask your health care provider if this type of exercise is OK for you.

- Drink plenty of water. Restricting fluid does not ease swelling, so drink up.

- Avoid excessive sodium. Sodium attracts water and helps your body to hold on to fluid.

- Focus on including enough fruits and vegetables in your eating plan. Produce is rich in potassium, a mineral that counteracts the effects of sodium and promotes better fluid balance that may reduce swelling.

FROM THE RECIPE FILE

Foods rich in potassium, such as Mashed Potatoes with Greens and Cheese (page 291), help to keep swelling to a minimum.

CONCLUSION

You've just read about some of the things that can go wrong in a pregnancy as well as some relatively minor discomforts. Chances are your pregnancy will turn out fine, even when complications such as diabetes or high blood pressure arise, because we know so much about how to treat pregnancy problems. Getting regular medical attention throughout your pregnancy, even when you feel good, is the best way to ensure that you'll have the healthiest baby possible.

If you've read this book from cover to cover, you've learned about the most recent evidence regarding the effects of a healthy lifestyle on your well-being as a parent and on your baby's health. Your own experiences during pregnancy and parenthood will add to what you've discovered here.

This is not the end of the road! The best is yet to come: an entire chapter devoted to delicious and nutritious recipes, followed by resources and references to explore. The main part of this book is finished, but it's just the beginning of a lifetime with your new baby. Enjoy every moment!

8

Quick and Delicious Recipes

Y̶ou're having a baby, trying to get pregnant, or breastfeeding. You want to eat delicious and nutritious food, but you don't always have the time to prepare it. Rest easy. *Expect the Best*'s healthy recipes taste great, use everyday ingredients, and require little fuss.

To make it easier to follow the eating recommendations discussed in *Expect the Best,* most of the recipes in this chapter call for lower-sodium and lower-fat versions of common ingredients, and the recipes keep added sugar to a minimum. However, nearly all the recipes are flexible, so use the ingredients that are right for you, and make the substitutions that work best for you and your family. For example, cooking spray, which is called for in some of the recipes, prevents food from sticking to the pan, but you can swap it for olive oil, canola oil, or any other type of fat, if you'd like.

Three types of symbols will help you to identify the recipes that are vegetarian, dairy-free, and gluten-free.

Vegetarian recipes contain no meat, poultry, or seafood, but they may have dairy products and eggs. However, some vegetarian recipes may also be completely free of animal products (vegan).

Dairy-free recipes contain no milk, cheese, yogurt, or other dairy products.

Gluten-free recipes don't include any ingredients with known sources of gluten.

Each recipe includes nutrition information per serving, and the amount of added sugar is listed in grams and in teaspoons. For more information on added sugar, see page 39.

You'll also find the food group amounts so you know how each portion fits into your MyPlate eating recommendations, which you can read about in chapter 3. Baby, let's eat!

BEVERAGES AND SMOOTHIE BOWLS

Smoothies and Smoothie Bowls

When you don't feel much like eating, and even when your appetite is good, healthy smoothies and smoothie bowls are an easy option for providing several of the nutrients you need. Many people start their day with smoothies or smoothie bowls, but you can enjoy them at any meal—and even as a snack.

Smoothie "Rules"

The first rule about smoothies is that there are very few rules to follow! However, the most balanced basic smoothie combines fruit or vegetables, or both, with protein- and calcium-rich foods, such as yogurt and milk. Using lower-fat dairy products as the basis of smoothies helps better control calories and saturated fat, but you can use whatever type of dairy works for you, or swap in unsweetened fortified soy beverages to make vegan smoothies. You may also use other plant-based milks, such as almond milk, but the protein content will be significantly lower.

Frozen produce makes for thicker smoothies and a more intense flavor because you don't have to use ice. Depending on the other ingredients in the smoothie, ice may dilute the drink. To freeze fresh fruit, wash and dry it thoroughly. Slice fruit such as strawberries, bananas, and peaches before freezing, place fruit on a baking sheet, and freeze for an hour. Transfer fruit to a freezer-safe bag or container and return to the freezer. You can also purchase plain frozen fruit.

Fresh and frozen fruit provides sweetness, especially when very ripe, and that helps to limit the amount of added sugar you need. Added sugar is relatively low, or absent from, all of *Expect the Best*'s recipes, so use sweeteners if desired, and if they fit within your eating plan.

BASIC SMOOTHIE RECIPE

Makes 1 serving. 🚫 🌾

1 cup fresh or frozen fruit or vegetables, or a combination

$1/2$ cup milk or unsweetened fortified soy beverage

$1/2$ cup plain Greek yogurt

Place the ingredients in a blender or food processor. Blend on high speed for 1 to 2 minutes, or until frothy. Pour into a tall glass and enjoy immediately.

You can customize smoothies and smoothie bowls to suit your taste. The flavor combinations are limited only by your imagination. You don't have to add anything to the basic smoothie recipe, but here's a list of possibilities and suggested amounts for beverages and smoothie bowls.

FOR MORE FIBER:

Chia seeds, 1–2 tablespoons

Hemp seeds, 1–2 tablespoons

Whole flaxseeds (grind just before using), 1 tablespoon

Sesame seeds, 1 tablespoon

Oats, uncooked, 2 tablespoons

FOR MORE PROTEIN:

Hemp protein powder, 2 tablespoons

Pea protein powder, 2 tablespoons

Peanut powder, 3 tablespoons

Chocolate protein powder,
3 tablespoons

Whey protein powder, plain,
3 tablespoons

Instant skim milk powder,
4 tablespoons

FOR MORE PHYTONUTRIENTS:

Kale, $1/2$ cup raw

Baby spinach, $1/2$ cup raw

Unsweetened cocoa powder,
1 tablespoon

FOR MORE FLAVOR:

Cinnamon, $1/8$ teaspoon

Ground cayenne pepper, pinch

Medjool dates, 5

FOR MORE HEALTHY FATS:

Almonds, 2 tablespoons

Avocado, $1/4$ whole

Cashews, 2 tablespoons

Hazelnuts, 2 tablespoons

Pecans, 2 tablespoons

Peanuts, 2 tablespoons

Pistachios, 2 tablespoons

Walnuts, 2 tablespoons

Almond butter, 1 tablespoon

Peanut butter, 1 tablespoon

Sunflower seed butter, 1 tablespoon

Tahini, 1 tablespoon

MAKE-AHEAD SMOOTHIES

Assemble and freeze smoothie ingredients ahead of time. It saves time, and you can make a different smoothie every day! Here's one example of a freezer smoothie kit: place $1/2$ cup blueberries, $1/2$ cup fresh, washed, and dried spinach, and 2 tablespoons uncooked oats in a freezer-friendly container or reusable bag. When you're ready, blend the kit ingredients with yogurt and milk.

CAFÉ AU LAIT

Makes 1 serving. 🍵 🌾

This delicious drink packs bone-building calcium and protein. Chill and serve it over ice for a change of pace.

1 cup 1% low-fat milk

2 teaspoons sugar or sweetener of your choice (optional)

1 cup hot, strong, brewed decaffeinated coffee

Ground cinnamon or unsweetened cocoa powder, if desired

In a small saucepan, heat the milk and sugar over medium heat until warm. Place the milk mixture in a blender or food processor. Blend on high speed until frothy (about 1 minute), or use a handheld frother. Pour half of the coffee into a mug, then add the frothed milk. Sprinkle with cinnamon or cocoa.

PER SERVING:

Calories: 133

Total fat: 2 grams

Saturated fat: 1 gram

Cholesterol: 12 milligrams

Sodium: 107 milligrams

Carbohydrate: 21 grams

Dietary fiber: 0

Protein: 8 grams

Calcium: 296 milligrams

Iron: 0

Added sugar: 8 grams; 2 teaspoons

MyPlate food groups:

Dairy: 1 cup

GINGER TEA

Makes 4 servings. 🫙 🌾 🍼

When you're queasy, ginger might help settle your stomach. Make a batch of ginger tea, and refrigerate for when morning sickness hits. Drink it warm or cold.

4 cups water

4-inch piece of gingerroot, peeled and roughly chopped

In a small saucepan over medium heat, bring the water and ginger to a boil, cover the pan, and simmer for 5 minutes. Remove the pan from heat, and allow the tea to sit for 5 minutes. Strain the tea or leave the gingerroot in for a more intense flavor. Sweeten as desired. Drink immediately or store in refrigerator.

PER SERVING:

Calories: 0

Total fat: 0

Saturated fat: 0

Cholesterol: 0

Sodium: 0

Carbohydrate: 0

Dietary fiber: 0

Protein: 0

Calcium: 0

Iron: 0

Added sugar: 0

MyPlate food groups:

None, but the tea counts toward your fluid requirements.

MOCHA JAVA SMOOTHIE
Makes 1 serving. 🌶 🌾

*Get the taste of the coffee you crave without all the caffeine,
and get a third of your daily vitamin D requirements, too.*

1 tablespoon warm water

1 teaspoon decaffeinated instant coffee granules

1 cup 1% low-fat milk

1 tablespoon fat-free chocolate syrup

2 teaspoons unsweetened cocoa powder

1 ice cube

In a small bowl, dissolve the coffee granules in the warm water, then place in a blender or food processor. Add the milk, chocolate syrup, cocoa powder, and ice. Blend on high speed for 1 to 2 minutes, or until frothy. Pour into a tall glass and enjoy immediately.

PER SERVING:

Calories: 157

Total fat: 3 grams

Saturated fat: 2 grams

Cholesterol: 12 milligrams

Sodium: 121 milligrams

Carbohydrate: 25 grams

Dietary fiber: 1 gram

Protein: 9 grams

Calcium: 296 milligrams

Iron: 1 milligram

Added sugar: 12 grams; 3 teaspoons

MyPlate food groups:

Dairy: 1 cup

CHOCOLATE BANANA BLAST

Makes 1 serving. 🍽 🌾

A calcium-rich beverage that combines a serving each of fruit and milk. Use a frozen banana for a frothier drink.

1 medium banana, peeled and sliced

1 cup 1% low-fat milk

1 tablespoon unsweetened cocoa powder

1 ice cube

Place the ingredients in a blender or food processor. Blend on high speed for 1 to 2 minutes, or until frothy. Pour into a tall glass and enjoy immediately.

PER SERVING:

Calories: 207

Total fat: 3 grams

Saturated fat: 2 grams

Cholesterol: 12 milligrams

Sodium: 109 milligrams

Carbohydrate: 40 grams

Dietary fiber: 3 grams

Protein: 10 grams

Calcium: 296 milligrams

Iron: 0

Added sugar: 0

MyPlate food groups:

Dairy: 1 cup

Fruit: 1 cup

BLUEBERRY-ORANGE-MANGO SMOOTHIE

Makes 1 serving. 🥤 🌾

Are you in the mood for something fruity? This smoothie is sure to tempt your taste buds. Use fortified orange juice for even more vitamins and minerals.

$1/2$ cup fresh or frozen unsweetened blueberries

$1/2$ cup fresh or frozen unsweetened mango

$1/2$ cup plain fat-free Greek yogurt

$3/4$ cup 100% orange juice

Place the ingredients in a blender or food processor. Blend on high speed for 1 to 2 minutes, or until frothy. Pour into a tall glass and drink immediately.

PER SERVING:

Calories: 247

Total fat: 1 gram

Saturated fat: 0

Cholesterol: 0

Sodium: 57 milligrams

Carbohydrate: 43 grams

Dietary fiber: 4 grams

Protein: 14 grams

Calcium: 185 milligrams

Iron: 0

Added sugar: 0

MyPlate food groups:

Fruit: $13/4$ cups

Dairy: $1/2$ cup

CHERRY VANILLA COOLER

Makes 1 serving. 🍖 🌾

*Cherries supply natural sweetness
plus beneficial fiber and phytonutrients.*

$1/2$ medium banana, peeled

$1/2$ cup frozen or fresh sweet cherries, no sugar added, pitted

$1/2$ cup plain fat-free Greek yogurt

1 teaspoon pure vanilla extract

1 tablespoon 1% low-fat milk

Place the banana in a blender or food processor and process on high speed until smooth. Add the cherries, yogurt, vanilla extract, and milk. Blend on high speed for 1 minute, or until frothy. Pour into a tall glass and drink immediately.

PER SERVING:

Calories: 196

Total fat: 1 gram

Saturated fat: 0

Cholesterol: 2 milligrams

Sodium: 49 milligrams

Carbohydrate: 37 grams

Dietary fiber: 4 grams

Protein: 10 grams

Calcium: 150 milligrams

Iron: 0

Added sugar: 0

MyPlate food groups:

Fruit: 1 cup

Dairy: $1/2$ cup

PUMPKIN PIE SMOOTHIE
Makes 1 serving.

*Drink your vegetables with this healthier
pumpkin pie alternative. You can make this
with cooked or canned sweet potato, too.*

3/4 cup 1% low-fat milk

1/2 cup plain canned pumpkin

2 teaspoons packed brown sugar (or less, or sweetener of your choice)

1 teaspoon pure vanilla extract

pinch each: ground cinnamon, ground nutmeg, ground cloves

2 ice cubes

Place the ingredients in a blender or food processor. Blend on high
speed for 1 to 2 minutes, or until frothy. Pour into a tall glass and drink
immediately.

PER SERVING:

Calories: 153

Total fat: 2 grams

Saturated fat: 1 gram

Cholesterol: 9 milligrams

Sodium: 89 milligrams

Carbohydrate: 28 grams

Dietary fiber: 4 grams

Protein: 8 grams

Calcium: 260 milligrams

Iron: 2 milligrams

Added sugar: 8 grams; 2 teaspoons

MyPlate food groups:

Dairy: 3/4 cup

Vegetable: 1/2 cup

STRAWBERRY PEACH SIPPER

Makes 1 serving. 🍳 🌾 🍼

This smoothie makes it a snap to include the protein, calcium, fiber, and other nutrients you need.

3/4 cup unsweetened fortified soy milk

1/2 cup frozen sliced unsweetened strawberries

1/2 cup frozen sliced unsweetened peaches

1/2 teaspoon pure vanilla extract

Place the ingredients in a blender or food processor. Blend on high speed for 1 to 2 minutes, or until frothy. Pour into a tall glass and drink immediately.

PER SERVING:

Calories: 129

Total fat: 3 grams

Saturated fat: 0

Cholesterol: 0

Sodium: 58 milligrams

Carbohydrate: 21 grams

Dietary fiber: 5 grams

Protein: 6 grams

Calcium: 250 milligrams

Iron: 2 milligrams

Added sugar: 0

MyPlate food groups:

Fruit: 1 cup

Dairy: 3/4 cup

PEANUT, RASPBERRY, BANANA, AND OATS SMOOTHIE BOWL

Makes 1 serving. 🚫 🌾*

*if certified gluten-free oats are used

Peanut powder, also known as peanut butter powder, provides protein with fewer calories and less fat than peanut butter, and intensifies the peanut flavor. Use really ripe bananas for more natural sweetness.

$1/2$ cup plain fat-free Greek yogurt

$1/4$ cup 1% low-fat milk

3 tablespoons peanut powder

1 medium frozen ripe banana, sliced

$1/4$ cup one-minute oats

$1/2$ teaspoon pure vanilla extract

Toppings

$1/2$ medium banana, chopped

$1/2$ cup fresh raspberries

2 tablespoons chopped peanuts

Place the yogurt, milk, peanut powder, banana, oats, and vanilla extract in a blender or food processor. Blend on high speed for 1 to 2 minutes, or until smooth. Pour into a cereal bowl. Arrange the sliced banana, raspberries, and peanuts on top.

PER SERVING:

Calories: 473

Total fat: 8 grams

Saturated fat: 1 gram

Cholesterol: 3 milligrams

Sodium: 140 milligrams

Carbohydrate: 70 grams

Dietary fiber: 13 grams

Protein: 29 grams

Calcium: 280 milligrams

Iron: 2 milligrams

Added sugar: 0

MyPlate food groups:

Fruit: 2 cups

Dairy: $3/4$ cup

Grain: $1/2$ ounce-equivalent (whole grain)

GO GREEN SMOOTHIE BOWL
Makes 1 serving. 🍳 🌾 🍼

This bowl is brimming with phytonutrients
that protect cells and fiber to keep you regular.
It's vegan, use cow's milk, if desired.

$^1/_2$ cup baby kale

$^1/_2$ medium frozen ripe banana, sliced

$^1/_2$ pitted avocado, sliced

$^1/_2$ cup unsweetened soy milk

Toppings

$^1/_2$ cup fresh pineapple slices or chunks, or canned in its own juice and drained

$^1/_2$ cup fresh sliced strawberries

2 tablespoons chia seeds

Place the kale, banana, avocado, and soy milk in a blender or food processor. Blend on high speed for 1 to 2 minutes, or until smooth. Pour into a cereal bowl.

Arrange the pineapple, strawberries, and chia seeds on top.

PER SERVING:

Calories: 417

Total fat: 22 grams

Saturated fat: 3 grams

Cholesterol: 0

Sodium: 64 milligrams

Carbohydrate: 53 grams

Dietary fiber: 18 grams

Protein: 10 grams

Calcium: 330 milligrams

Iron: 2 milligrams

Added sugar: 0

MyPlate food groups:

Fruit: 1$^1/_2$ cups

Vegetable: 1 cup

Dairy: $^1/_2$ cup

JOY OF ALMOND
SMOOTHIE BOWL

Makes 1 serving. 🚫 🌾

Who needs a candy bar when you've got this to enjoy? Swap mini chocolate chips for slivered almonds to satisfy a chocolate craving!

1/2 medium frozen ripe banana, sliced

1/2 cup plain fat-free Greek yogurt

1 tablespoon natural almond butter

2 teaspoons unsweetened cocoa powder

1/2 teaspoon pure vanilla extract

Toppings:

1 tablespoon unsweetened coconut

1/2 chopped banana

2 tablespoons slivered almonds

Place the banana, yogurt, almond butter, cocoa powder, and vanilla extract in a blender or food processor. Blend on high speed for 1 to 2 minutes, or until smooth. Pour into a cereal bowl.

Arrange the coconut, chopped banana, and almonds on top.

PER SERVING:

Calories: 409

Total fat: 22 grams

Saturated fat: 9 grams

Cholesterol: 0

Sodium: 131 milligrams

Carbohydrate: 35 grams

Dietary fiber: 7 grams

Protein: 18 grams

Calcium: 220 milligrams

Iron: 1 milligram

Added sugar: 0

MyPlate food groups:

Fruit: 1 cup

Dairy: 1/2 cup

BREAKFAST

EGG AND VEGETABLE WRAP
Makes 1 serving. 🚫 💊

Good things come in small packages. Eggs are a good source of protein, vitamin D, and riboflavin (a B vitamin), and an excellent source of choline. Eggs are for any time of the day. You don't need to wait for breakfast to enjoy this wrap!

2 large eggs

2 tablespoons water

$1/4$ cup diced red bell pepper or cooked broccoli, asparagus, or mushrooms

1 7-inch whole-wheat tortilla

In a small bowl, beat together the eggs and water. Coat a 7-inch omelet pan with cooking spray and heat over medium-high heat. When the pan is hot, pour in the egg mixture. Gently pull in the sides of the egg mixture with a small rubber spatula, and tilt the pan to move the egg around until it covers the pan. When no visible liquid egg remains, sprinkle the top of the egg with vegetables. Place the tortilla on a plate. Carefully slide the egg onto the tortilla. Roll up, and enjoy with salsa, if desired.

PER SERVING (WITHOUT THE SALSA):

Calories: 229

Total fat: 11 grams

Saturated fat: 3 grams

Cholesterol: 423 milligrams

Sodium: 290 milligrams

Carbohydrate: 19 grams

Dietary fiber: 3 grams

Protein: 16 grams

Calcium: 60 milligrams

Iron: 3 milligrams

Added sugar: 0, unless the tortilla contains some.

MyPlate food groups:

Grain: 1 ounce-equivalent (whole grain)

Protein: 2 ounce-equivalents

Vegetable: $1/4$ cup

AVOCADO STUFFED WITH EGG, CHEESE, AND SALSA

Makes 2 servings. 🚫 🌾

The combination of the protein in the egg and the cheese and the healthy fat and fiber in the avocado will keep you satisfied for hours.

2 large eggs

$1/4$ cup shredded reduced-fat cheddar cheese

1 ripe avocado, cut lengthwise and pitted

2 tablespoons salsa without added sugar

Freshly ground black pepper

Coat a medium nonstick skillet with cooking spray. Heat over medium heat.

Beat the eggs in a small bowl. Add the cheese. Pour the egg mixture into the skillet and scramble.

Place half the cooked egg mixture in each of the cavities in the avocado halves. Top each half with 1 tablespoon of the salsa, and add freshly ground black pepper, if desired.

PER SERVING:

Calories: 265

Total fat: 21 grams

Saturated fat: 4 grams

Cholesterol: 215 milligrams

Sodium: 274 milligrams

Carbohydrate: 10 grams

Fiber: 7 grams

Protein: 13 grams

Calcium: 111 milligrams

Iron: 2 milligrams

Added sugar: 0

MyPlate food groups:

Dairy: $1/3$ cup

Protein: 2 ounce-equivalents

Vegetable: $1/2$ cup

OVERNIGHT PINEAPPLE KIWI BREAKFAST PARFAIT

Makes 2 servings. (🚫) (🌾)*

*if certified gluten-free oats are used

Make this energizing parfait in a mason jar tonight and enjoy a healthy, easy breakfast tomorrow morning.

2/3 cup old-fashioned oats, uncooked

1 tablespoon honey or pure maple syrup

1 teaspoon pure vanilla extract

1 1/2 cups plain fat-free Greek yogurt

2 kiwi, peeled and cubed

1/2 cup fresh (or canned and drained) pineapple chunks

In a small bowl, combine the oats with the honey, vanilla extract, and yogurt.

Divide half the oat mixture evenly between two half-pint mason jars (reserve the remaining half for the next layer). In a small bowl, combine the kiwi and pineapple. Layer half of the fruit mixture on top of the oat mixture. Add the remaining oat mixture and the fruit. Cover and refrigerate overnight.

PER SERVING:

Calories: 269

Total fat: 2 gram

Saturated fat: 0

Cholesterol: 7 milligrams

Sodium: 136 milligrams

Carbohydrate: 41 grams

Dietary fiber: 5 grams

Protein: 21 grams

Calcium: 250 milligrams

Iron: 7 milligrams

Added sugar: 8 grams; 2 teaspoons

MyPlate food groups:

Dairy: 3/4 cup

Grain: 1 ounce-equivalent (whole grain)

Fruit: 1 cup

FRUIT AND NUT BREAD

Makes 12 servings. *

*if certified gluten-free oats are used

You don't have to use two types of nuts and dried fruit to make this no-added-sugar delight. Use whatever dried fruits and nuts you have in the house.

2 medium ripe bananas, broken into large chunks

2 large eggs

1/4 cup canola oil

2 cups oat flour*

1 teaspoon baking powder

1/2 teaspoon salt

3/4 cup chopped almonds

3/4 cup chopped walnuts

3/4 cup dried unsweetened apricots, chopped

3/4 cup raisins

Preheat the oven to 350°F.

Coat a 1 1/2-quart loaf pan with cooking spray, and line with a sheet of parchment paper.

In a large mixing bowl, mash the bananas until no longer chunky. Using a whisk, add the eggs and oil and combine well.

Add the oat flour, baking powder, and salt. Stir to combine. Add the almonds, walnuts, apricots, and raisins, and blend well.

Pour the batter into the loaf pan and spread the batter evenly.

Bake for 25 to 30 minutes or until a toothpick inserted in the middle comes out clean.

*To make oat flour, place 2 cups of one-minute or old-fashioned oats in the food processor, and process on high speed until oats achieve a powder-like consistency, about 1 minute.

PER SERVING (1 SLICE OR $1/_{12}$ OF THE LOAF):

Calories: 253

Total fat: 14 grams

Saturated fat: 1 gram

Cholesterol: 35 milligrams

Sodium: 153 milligrams

Carbohydrate: 29 grams

Dietary fiber: 4 grams

Protein: 6 grams

Calcium: 64 milligrams

Iron: 2 milligrams

Added sugar: 0

MyPlate food groups:

Grain: $3/_4$ ounce-equivalent
(whole grain)

QUINOA BREAKFAST COOKIES
Makes 3 large cookies. 🚫 🌾 🥛

Pair one of these protein-rich breakfast goodies with a glass of low-fat milk and a piece of fruit for a balanced morning meal.

1 cup cooked red quinoa

$1/_2$ cup peanut butter

3 tablespoons peanut powder

1 tablespoon honey

In a medium bowl, combine the quinoa, peanut butter, peanut powder, and honey. Form into 3 balls, and flatten each into a cookie shape. Refrigerate.

PER SERVING (1 COOKIE):

Calories: 371

Total fat: 24 grams

Saturated fat: 5 grams

Cholesterol: 0

Sodium: 202 milligrams

Carbohydrate: 29 grams

Dietary fiber: 5 grams

Protein: 16 grams

Calcium: 36 milligrams

Iron: 2 milligrams

Added sugar: 6 grams; $1^1/_2$ teaspoons sugar

MyPlate food groups:

Grain: 1 ounce-equivalent
(whole grain)

WALNUT RAISIN MUFFINS
Makes 24 muffins.

These healthier muffins are great for breakfast on the run, and they make for a delicious snack, too.

2 cups all-purpose flour

1 cup whole-wheat flour

1 tablespoon baking powder

1 tablespoon ground cinnamon

1 teaspoon salt

1 teaspoon baking soda

1 cup one-minute oats, uncooked

$3/4$ cup light brown sugar, packed

1 cup raisins

1 cup chopped walnuts

$2^1/2$ cups unsweetened applesauce

$2/3$ cup canola oil

4 large eggs

$1/2$ cup 1% low-fat milk

Preheat the oven to 350°F. Line a 24-cup muffin pan with paper baking cups.

In a large mixing bowl, combine the all-purpose flour, whole-wheat flour, baking powder, cinnamon, salt, baking soda, oats, brown sugar, raisins, and walnuts. Stir until well combined.

Place the applesauce, oil, eggs, and milk in the bowl of an electric mixer. Blend on high speed until combined, about 1 minute.

Add the applesauce mixture to the flour mixture. Stir until the dry ingredients are just moistened.

Fill each muffin cup about $3/4$ full with batter. Bake for 12 to 15 minutes or until a toothpick inserted in the center of a muffin comes out clean. Remove the muffins from the pans and cool on a wire rack.

PER SERVING (1 MUFFIN):

Calories: 226

Total fat: 11 grams

Saturated fat: 1 gram

Cholesterol: 36 milligrams

Sodium: 227 milligrams

Carbohydrate: 30 grams

Dietary fiber: 2 grams

Protein: 4 grams

Calcium: 62 milligrams

Iron: 2 milligrams

Added sugar: 7 grams; nearly 2 level teaspoons

MyPlate food groups:

Grain: 2 ounce-equivalents

SPINACH, RED BELL PEPPER, AND CHEESE CUPS

Makes 6 servings. 🍳 🌾

It's hard to believe that so much great taste and good nutrition can be packed into such a portable snack or starter to your day! Enjoy with a slice of whole-grain toast and fruit for a balanced meal or hearty snack.

1 teaspoon olive oil

$1/2$ medium onion, chopped

$1/2$ medium red bell pepper, chopped

1 cup low-fat cottage cheese

2 large eggs

9-ounce package plain frozen chopped spinach, defrosted and well-drained

1 cup shredded Swiss cheese or other hard cheese

$1/4$ teaspoon fresh ground black pepper

Preheat oven to 400°F.

Coat 6 muffin cups with cooking spray.

In a small skillet, heat the oil over medium heat. Add the onions and bell pepper. Sauté for 5 minutes.

Place the cottage cheese in a food processor. Blend until smooth, about 45 seconds. Set aside. In a large bowl, whisk the eggs until just beaten. Add the cottage cheese, onions and peppers, spinach, cheese, and black pepper to the eggs. Mix well.

Divide the egg mixture evenly among the 6 muffin cups. Bake until firm, about 20 minutes. Remove from the oven and place on a wire cooling rack for 5 minutes. Remove from the pan and cool for 5 more minutes.

PER SERVING:

Calories: 146

Total fat: 8 grams

Saturated fat: 4 grams

Cholesterol: 89 milligrams

Sodium: 247 milligrams

Carbohydrate: 6 grams

Dietary fiber: 2 grams

Protein: 14 grams

Calcium: 240 milligrams

Iron: 1 milligram

Added sugar: 0

MyPlate food groups:

Dairy: $1/2$ cup

Vegetable: $1/4$ cup

ALMOND-FLOUR PANCAKES
WITH SMASHED RASPBERRIES
Makes 4 servings. 🚫 🌾

*One portion provides more than half the vitamin E and
over 25 percent of the fiber you need for the day, along
with several other nutrients. Cool any leftover pancakes
completely, freeze in a single layer on a baking sheet,
wrap, and store in the freezer for future meals or snacks.*

$1^1/_2$ cups almond flour or almond meal

$^1/_2$ teaspoon baking soda

$^1/_4$ teaspoon salt

3 large eggs

$^1/_4$ cup 1% low-fat milk

1 tablespoon pure maple syrup

1 tablespoon canola oil

1 teaspoon pure vanilla extract

$^1/_4$ teaspoon lemon juice

2 cups frozen raspberries

In a medium bowl, combine the almond flour, baking soda, and salt. In
another medium bowl, whisk together the eggs, milk, maple syrup, oil,
vanilla extract, and lemon juice. Add the egg mixture to the almond-
flour mixture and stir until just combined.

Coat a griddle or large skillet with cooking spray and heat over medium
heat. Drop pancake batter by scant $^1/_4$-cup portions onto the griddle,
and spread to form 4-inch round pancakes.

Cook for about 3 minutes or until pancakes begin to brown around the
edges and form bubbles in the middle. Do not overcook. Flip and cook
for another minute.

Place frozen raspberries in a microwave-safe bowl. Cover and micro-wave on high for 30 to 45 seconds. Mash with a fork to break up into smaller chunks. Drain excess fluid, if desired. If using fresh raspberries, mash lightly or use whole. To serve, top pancakes with raspberries.

PER SERVING (2 PANCAKES):

Calories: 341

Total fat: 25 grams

Saturated fat: 3 grams

Cholesterol: 159 milligrams

Sodium: 360 milligrams

Carbohydrate: 19 grams

Dietary fiber: 8 grams

Protein: 14 grams

Calcium: 151 milligrams

Iron: 3 milligrams

Added sugar: 3 grams; about 1 teaspoon

MyPlate food groups:

Protein: 2 ounce-equivalents

Fruit: $1/2$ cup

BLUEBERRY BANANA PANCAKES

Makes 1 serving. 🚫 🌾 🥛

For a more intense taste, try to use fresh wild blueberries in this gluten-free pancake recipe, but if you can't, frozen will do just fine!

1 medium ripe banana

2 large eggs

$1/2$ teaspoon pure vanilla extract (optional)

2 teaspoons canola oil

$1/2$ cup blueberries

Break the banana into large chunks and place in a medium bowl. Using a fork, thoroughly mash the banana until it's nearly smooth and without large lumps.

In a small bowl, whisk the eggs with the vanilla extract. Add the egg mixture to the mashed banana and stir until combined.

Heat the oil in a large skillet or griddle over medium heat. Drop the batter in about $1/4$-cup portions onto the skillet to make 2 pancakes. Cook for 1 minute. Sprinkle the blueberries on top of the batter. Carefully flip the pancakes (they are more delicate than regular pancakes), and cook for another minute or until browned.

PER SERVING:

Calories: 367

Total fat: 20 grams

Saturated fat: 4 grams

Cholesterol: 423 milligrams

Sodium: 142 milligrams

Carbohydrate: 37 grams

Dietary fiber: 5 grams

Protein: 14 grams

Calcium: 65 milligrams

Iron: 2 milligrams

Added sugar: 0

MyPlate food groups:

Protein: 2 ounce-equivalents

Fruit: $1^1/2$ cups

TOAST THREE WAYS

Each recipe makes 1 serving.

Whole-grain toast is a staple of the morning meal, and it's even better for you when paired with protein. Blend cottage cheese in a food processor and keep it on hand to make tempting toast combinations for breakfast or for snacks. For less sodium, use no-added-salt cottage cheese. You can also use ricotta cheese in place of cottage cheese.

STRAWBERRY BALSAMIC TOAST

2-ounces whole-grain toast 🚫

$1/4$ cup low-fat cottage cheese

$1/2$ cup chopped fresh strawberries

1 teaspoon balsamic vinegar

Salt and freshly ground black pepper (optional)

Spread the cottage cheese on the toast. Layer with the strawberries and drizzle with the vinegar. Add salt and pepper, if desired.

PER SERVING:

Calories: 218

Total fat: 3 grams

Saturated fat: 1 gram

Cholesterol: 2 milligrams

Sodium: 522 milligrams

Carbohydrate: 33 grams

Dietary fiber: 6 grams

Protein: 16 grams

Calcium: 112 milligrams

Iron: 2 milligrams

Added sugar: 0

MyPlate food groups:

Grain: 2 ounce-equivalents (whole grain)

Fruit: $1/2$ cup

Dairy: $1/4$ cup

MAPLE, PECAN, AND APPLE TOAST

2-ounces whole-grain toast 🚫

$1/4$ cup low-fat cottage cheese

$1/2$ apple, sliced

2 tablespoons chopped pecans

1 teaspoon pure maple syrup

Spread the cottage cheese on the toast. Layer with the apple and the pecans, and drizzle the maple syrup on top.

PER SERVING:

Calories: 458

Total fat: 16 grams

Saturated fat: 2 grams

Cholesterol: 2 milligrams

Sodium: 551 milligrams

Carbohydrate: 68 grams

Dietary fiber: 9 grams

Protein: 16 grams

Calcium: 84 milligrams

Iron: 4 milligrams

Added sugar: 4 grams; 1 teaspoon

MyPlate food groups:

Grain: 2 ounce-equivalents (whole grain)

Fruit: $1/2$ cup

Dairy: $1/4$ cup

HONEY-PEAR WALNUT TOAST

2-ounces whole-grain toast 🍽

$1/4$ cup low-fat cottage cheese

$1/2$ pear, sliced

2 tablespoons chopped walnuts

1 teaspoon honey

Spread the cottage cheese on the toast. Layer with the pear and the walnuts, and drizzle the honey on top.

PER SERVING:

Calories: 358

Total fat: 12 grams

Saturated fat: 2 grams

Cholesterol: 2 milligrams

Sodium: 522 milligrams

Carbohydrate: 49 grams

Dietary fiber: 8 grams

Protein: 18 grams

Calcium: 122 milligrams

Iron: 2 milligrams

Added sugar: 6 grams; $1^1/2$ teaspoons

MyPlate food groups:

Grain: 2 ounce-equivalents (whole grain)

Fruit: $1/2$ cup

Dairy: $1/4$ cup

ENTREES

CHICKEN WITH WHOLE-WHEAT COUSCOUS, CRANBERRIES, AND ALMONDS

Makes 2 servings. 🍶

Whole-wheat couscous has more fiber, vitamins, and minerals than regular couscous. Farro and freekeh are nutritious couscous substitutes.

1$\frac{1}{4}$ cups low-sodium chicken broth, divided

$\frac{1}{2}$ cup whole-wheat couscous, uncooked

2 teaspoons olive oil

1 small onion, peeled and sliced thin

8 ounces boneless, skinless chicken breast, cut in $\frac{1}{2}$-inch cubes

2 cloves garlic, peeled and diced

$\frac{1}{4}$ teaspoon ground cumin

$\frac{1}{4}$ teaspoon ground ginger

$\frac{1}{4}$ teaspoon ground cinnamon

1 cup finely grated peeled carrots

$\frac{1}{3}$ cup dried sweetened cranberries

$\frac{1}{4}$ cup slivered almonds

In a small saucepan, bring $\frac{3}{4}$ cup of the chicken broth to a boil. Add the couscous. Cover and let stand for five minutes. Remove from heat and set aside.

Meanwhile, in a large skillet, heat the oil over medium-high heat. Add the onion and sauté until clear, about 3 minutes. Add the chicken and cook, stirring, until lightly browned, about 5 minutes. Add the remaining $\frac{1}{2}$ cup chicken broth, garlic, cumin, ginger, and cinnamon. Simmer over low heat until the meat is cooked through, about 5 to 7 minutes.

Place the cooked couscous in a large serving bowl. Add the chicken mixture and stir. Add the carrots and cranberries and mix well. Sprinkle with the almonds just before serving.

PER SERVING:

Calories: 400

Total fat: 11 grams

Saturated fat: 2 grams

Cholesterol: 57 milligrams

Sodium: 151 milligrams

Carbohydrate: 48 grams

Dietary fiber: 6 grams

Protein: 32 grams

Calcium: 70 milligrams

Iron: 3 milligrams

Added sugar: 12 grams; 3 teaspoons (from the sweetened cranberries)

MyPlate food groups:

Protein: 5 ounce-equivalents

Grain: 1 ounce-equivalent (whole grain)

Vegetable: 1 cup

SLOW-COOKER THAI PEANUT CHICKEN

Makes 4 servings. 🐦

You can substitute sunflower seed butter for the peanut butter. Serve with cooked jasmine rice, steamed green beans, and sliced mango.

16 ounces boneless, skinless chicken thighs

1/2 teaspoon freshly ground black pepper

3/4 cup mild tomato salsa without added sugar

1/3 cup smooth natural peanut butter

2 tablespoons lime juice

1 tablespoon reduced-sodium soy sauce

2 teaspoons peeled grated fresh ginger

1/4 cup chopped fresh cilantro (optional)

lime wedges (optional)

Season both sides of the chicken with the black pepper. Place the chicken in a slow cooker.

In a medium bowl, combine the salsa, peanut butter, lime juice, soy sauce, and ginger. Stir well. Pour over the chicken.

Cover the slow cooker and cook on low heat for 8 hours. Using a slotted spoon, remove the chicken from the slow cooker. Place on a serving platter. Remove the sauce from the slow cooker and pour over the chicken. Garnish with cilantro and lime wedges, if desired.

PER SERVING:

Calories: 274

Total fat: 15 grams

Saturated fat: 3 grams

Cholesterol: 93 milligrams

Sodium: 619 milligrams

Carbohydrate: 8 grams

Dietary fiber: 2 grams

Protein: 28 grams

Calcium: 34 milligrams

Iron: 2 milligrams

Added sugar: 0

MyPlate food groups:

Protein: 4 ounce-equivalents

BEEF WITH SNOW PEAS

Makes 4 servings. 🍶

The ginger and garlic sauce lends flavor to the meat and vegetables. Use any vegetables you have on hand. You can also substitute chicken, pork tenderloin, or tofu for the beef.

1/4 cup low-sodium soy sauce

2 tablespoons rice wine vinegar

2 tablespoons tomato paste

1 tablespoon packed brown sugar

4 cloves garlic, peeled and minced, or 2 teaspoons prepared minced garlic

2 teaspoons grated fresh ginger

1/4 teaspoon freshly ground black pepper

16 ounces boneless top round steak, trimmed of fat and sliced into 1/4-inch-by-1-inch pieces

1 tablespoon canola oil

1 1/2 cups fresh snow peas, chopped in half

1 5-ounce can sliced water chestnuts, drained

In a medium bowl, whisk together the soy sauce, vinegar, tomato paste, brown sugar, garlic, and ginger until well combined. Set aside.

Season the meat with the black pepper.

Heat the oil over medium-high heat in a wok or large skillet. When hot, add the beef and cook for 5 minutes. When the beef is cooked, lower the heat to medium, and add the soy sauce mixture. Toss to coat the beef completely. Add the snow peas and water chestnuts. Continue to cook, tossing constantly, for another 2 minutes. Serve warm.

PER SERVING:

Calories: 277

Total fat: 8 grams

Saturated fat: 2 grams

Cholesterol: 59 milligrams

Sodium: 644 milligrams

Carbohydrate: 16 grams

Dietary fiber: 2 grams

Protein: 34 grams

Calcium: 30 milligrams

Iron: 4 milligrams

Added sugar: 3 grams; almost 1 teaspoon

MyPlate food groups:

Protein: 4 ounce-equivalents

Vegetable: 1/2 cup

BAKED SPAGHETTI SQUASH CARBONARA

Makes 4 servings.

This squash dish mimics the flavors found in spaghetti carbonara. Cottage cheese jacks up the protein, so it's more than a side dish. Skip the bacon bits to make it vegetarian.

2 teaspoons olive oil

1 small yellow onion, diced

1 cup low-fat plain cottage cheese

1 tablespoon 1% low-fat milk

4 large eggs

$3/4$ cup grated Parmesan cheese, divided

$1/4$ cup reduced-fat bacon bits

$1/2$ teaspoon freshly ground black pepper

5 to 6 cups cooked spaghetti squash, well drained*

Preheat the oven to 350°F. Coat a 3-quart baking dish with cooking spray.

In a small skillet, heat the oil over medium heat. Add the onions and sauté until nearly clear, about 4 to 5 minutes. Set aside.

Place the cottage cheese in a blender or food processor with the milk. Blend until smooth, about 1 minute. Set aside.

In a large mixing bowl, whisk the eggs. Add the cottage cheese mixture and combine well. Add $1/2$ cup of the Parmesan cheese, the bacon, and the black pepper, and stir. Add the squash, and toss well to combine.

Pour the squash mixture into the baking dish, and sprinkle the top evenly with the remaining $1/4$ cup of Parmesan cheese. Bake for 20 to 25 minutes or until just firm.

*To cook the squash, split a 4- to 5-pound spaghetti squash lengthwise. Scoop out the seeds. Place each half of the squash face down in a microwavable dish. Add $1/4$ inch of water to the bottom of the dish. Cover, and microwave the squash on high for 15 to 20 minutes or until fork-tender. Repeat with the other half of the squash. When cool enough to handle, remove the squash from the dish. Flip it over to allow it to cool. Shred the squash with a fork into spaghetti-like strings, and remove from the shell. Drain. You can cook the squash up to three days ahead of time and refrigerate until ready to use.

PER SERVING:

Calories: 311

Total fat: 15 grams

Saturated fat: 7 grams

Cholesterol: 235 milligrams

Sodium: 866 milligrams

Carbohydrate: 20 grams

Dietary fiber: 4 grams

Protein: 25 grams

Calcium: 320 milligrams

Iron: 2 milligrams

Added sugar: 0

MyPlate food groups:

Vegetable: 1 cup

Dairy: $1/2$ cup

ARTICHOKE QUICHE WITH THYME AND GRUYERE CHEESE

Makes 6 servings. 🚫 🌾

If you're not a big milk drinker, you'll appreciate that this entrée supplies more than a third of your daily calcium needs. Swap in cooked broccoli if you're not a fan of artichokes.

1 tablespoon canola oil

1 medium onion, peeled and chopped

4 large eggs

1 12-ounce can evaporated milk

1 teaspoon dried thyme

1/4 teaspoon freshly ground black pepper

1 1/2 cup shredded Gruyere cheese, divided

1 cup quartered canned artichokes, drained and roughly chopped

Preheat the oven to 350°F. Lightly coat a 9-inch pie plate with cooking spray.

In a medium skillet, heat the oil over medium heat. Add the onions and sauté until nearly clear, about 4 to 5 minutes. Set aside.

In a medium mixing bowl, whisk together the eggs, evaporated milk, thyme, and black pepper.

Sprinkle 1/2 cup of the cheese into the pie plate. Top with the onions and the artichokes.

Pour the egg mixture into the pie plate. Sprinkle with the remaining cheese.

Bake for 30 to 35 minutes, or until a knife inserted in the center comes out clean. Cool on a wire rack for 10 minutes before serving.

PER SERVING:

Calories: 286

Total fat: 19 grams

Saturated fat: 9 grams

Cholesterol: 189 milligrams

Sodium: 222 milligrams

Carbohydrate: 12 grams

Dietary fiber: 3 grams

Protein: 18 grams

Calcium: 465 milligrams

Iron: 1 milligram

Added sugar: 0

MyPlate food groups:

Protein: 3 ounce-equivalents

Dairy: $1^1/_2$ cups

Vegetable: $^1/_4$ cup

SWEET BELL PEPPERS STUFFED WITH TOMATOES, RICE, AND CHEESE

Makes 3 servings. 🦐 🌾

Bell peppers are rich in vitamin C. Use wild or brown rice to include whole grains and fiber. Serve with a simple salad and fruit.

3 large red, yellow, or orange bell peppers, sliced in half lengthwise and cleaned of stems, seeds, and membranes

1 teaspoon olive oil

$1/2$ medium onion, peeled and chopped

1 cup cooked rice

1 cup canned no-salt-added stewed diced tomatoes, not drained

1 tablespoon tomato paste

2 teaspoons dried basil

$1/4$ teaspoon freshly ground black pepper

$1/2$ cup low-fat cottage cheese

$3/4$ cup shredded reduced-fat cheddar cheese or other hard cheese

Chopped fresh parsley for garnish, if desired

Preheat the oven to 350°F.

Bring 2 quarts of water to a boil in a large covered saucepan. Add the peppers, and boil for 3 to 5 minutes. Remove the peppers with a slotted spoon, pour the excess water from the pan, and return the peppers to the pan.

In a small nonstick skillet, heat the oil over medium heat. Add the onions and sauté until nearly clear, about 4 to 5 minutes.

Transfer the onions to a large bowl. Add the rice, tomatoes with their juice, tomato paste, basil, black pepper, and cottage cheese, and stir to combine.

Place the peppers cut side up in 9 x 13–inch baking dish. Spoon the cottage cheese and rice mixture into the pepper shells, dividing evenly. Top each pepper with equal amounts of cheddar cheese. Bake for 25 minutes or until heated through.

PER SERVING:

Calories: 230

Total fat: 5 grams

Saturated fat: 2 grams

Cholesterol: 7 milligrams

Sodium: 385 milligrams

Carbohydrate: 32 grams

Dietary fiber: 5 grams

Protein: 16 grams

Calcium: 190 milligrams

Iron: 3 milligrams

Added sugar: 0

MyPlate food groups:

Vegetable: 1 cup

Grain: 1 ounce-equivalent

Dairy: $3/4$ cup

SLOW-COOKER SPINACH LASAGNA

Makes 6 servings. 🚫

There's nothing better than knowing that a delicious and comforting meal is waiting for you at the end of your day.

1 24-ounce jar plus 1 cup marinara sauce

1 (14.5 ounce) can no-salt-added diced tomatoes, not drained

$1/4$ to $1/2$ teaspoon crushed red pepper, if desired

1 large yellow bell pepper, chopped into $1/2$-inch pieces

9 uncooked lasagna noodles

$1^1/2$ cups low-fat ricotta cheese

2 cups shredded part-skim mozzarella cheese

5 ounces coarsely chopped fresh baby spinach

Spray a 5- to 6-quart slow cooker with cooking spray. In a medium bowl, combine the marinara sauce, tomatoes, crushed red pepper, and bell pepper. Spread 1 cup of this mixture evenly in the bottom of the slow cooker.

Place 3 lasagna noodles, broken into pieces to fit, over the sauce in the slow cooker. Spread half of the ricotta cheese over the noodles, and sprinkle with $1/4$ cup of the mozzarella cheese and half of the spinach. Top with a third of the tomato sauce mixture (about $1^1/2$ cups).

Repeat the layering of the noodles, cheeses, and spinach. Top with the remaining 3 noodles and the remaining sauce. Set aside the remaining mozzarella cheese in the refrigerator.

Cover the slow cooker. Cook on low heat for about four hours or until the noodles are tender. Uncover slow cooker and sprinkle remaining mozzarella cheese on top. Cover and let sit for at least 5 minutes before serving.

PER SERVING:

Calories: 512

Total fat: 17 grams

Saturated fat: 9 grams

Cholesterol: 42 milligrams

Sodium: 926 milligrams

Carbohydrate: 62 grams

Dietary fiber: 7 grams

Protein: 26 grams

Calcium: 531 milligrams

Iron: 4 milligrams

Added sugar: Tomatoes contain some natural sugars, so the grams of sugar listed on the Nutrient Facts panel of any tomato product will not be zero. Purchase marinara sauce containing 7 grams or less of sugars per serving to be sure no sugar has been added.

MyPlate food groups:

Vegetable: $1^1/_2$ cups

Dairy: $1^1/_2$ cups

Grain: 1 ounce-equivalent

MACARONI AND CHEESE WITH BUTTERNUT SQUASH
Makes 6 servings. 🍽

This sophisticated version of a kid favorite will please the entire family. Use whole-wheat pasta for more fiber, if you like.

8 ounces (2 cups) elbow macaroni, uncooked

1 tablespoon canola oil

2 medium onions, peeled and chopped

3 cups (12 ounces) shredded reduced-fat sharp cheddar cheese or other hard cheese

1 tablespoon dried parsley

1/2 teaspoon dry mustard

1/2 teaspoon freshly ground black pepper

2 cups low-fat cottage cheese

1 cup pureed cooked butternut squash, thawed if frozen

1/4 cup 1% low-fat milk

1/4 cup plain bread crumbs

1/4 cup shredded Parmesan cheese

Preheat the oven to 350°F. Spray a 2-quart baking dish with cooking spray and set aside.

Cook the macaroni according to the package directions. Drain well and set aside.

In a small skillet, heat the oil over medium heat. Add the onions and sauté until they are nearly clear, about 4 to 5 minutes. Set aside.

In a large bowl, combine the cooked, drained macaroni, onions, cheddar cheese, parsley, mustard, and black pepper. Set aside.

Place the cottage cheese, squash, and milk in a food processor or a blender. Blend until smooth, about 45 seconds. Pour this mixture into the bowl with the macaroni and mix well. Pour the entire mixture into the baking dish.

In a small bowl, combine the bread crumbs and Parmesan cheese. Sprinkle evenly over the top of the macaroni mixture. Bake for about 30 minutes or until bubbly around the edges.

PER SERVING:

Calories: 373

Total fat: 9 grams

Saturated fat: 4 grams

Cholesterol: 19 milligrams

Sodium: 757 milligrams

Carbohydrate: 41 grams

Dietary fiber: 2 grams

Protein: 31 grams

Calcium: 370 milligrams

Iron: 2 milligrams

Added sugar: 0

MyPlate food groups:

Grain: 2 ounce-equivalents

Dairy: 1 cup

LINGUINE WITH ROASTED RED BELL PEPPER SAUCE

Makes 2 servings. 🚫 🍼

Tofu is the secret protein-boosting ingredient in this brightly colored entrée. Possible additions include 2 cups cooked chopped broccoli or 1 cup shredded cooked chicken.

4 ounces linguine, uncooked

1 cup jarred and drained roasted red bell peppers (2 large peppers)

$1/2$ cup silken tofu processed with calcium sulfate

$1^1/_2$ teaspoons jarred minced garlic

1 teaspoon fresh chopped thyme

$3/_4$ teaspoon salt

Cook linguine according to directions.

Place the red bell peppers, tofu, and garlic in a food processor and process on high speed until smooth, about 2 minutes. Transfer the red pepper mixture to a small saucepan. Add the thyme and salt, and warm the sauce for about 3 minutes.

Place the warm pasta in a serving bowl. Add the red pepper sauce and toss. Serve warm.

PER SERVING:

Calories: 214

Total fat: 6 grams

Saturated fat: 1 gram

Cholesterol: 0

Sodium: 884 milligrams

Carbohydrate: 28 grams

Dietary fiber: 3 grams

Protein: 14 grams

Calcium: 443 milligrams

Iron: 3 milligrams

Added sugar: 0

MyPlate food groups:

Grain: 2 ounce-equivalents

Vegetable: $1/2$ cup

SHRIMP, PINEAPPLE, AND ASPARAGUS STIR-FRY

Makes 2 servings. 🚫🍼

*Keep frozen shrimp on hand to make this
meal in a flash on a busy weeknight.*

1 tablespoon canola oil

$1/2$ medium onion, peeled and chopped

$1/2$ cup chopped red bell pepper

1 cup raw asparagus (about 12 stalks), washed,
ends trimmed, chopped into 1-inch lengths

3 cloves garlic, peeled and minced

8 ounces large raw shrimp, peeled and cleaned, defrosted if frozen

1 tablespoon reduced-sodium soy sauce

$1/2$ cup pineapple chunks, canned in their own juice, drained

In a large skillet, heat the oil over medium-high heat. Add the onions, peppers, garlic, and asparagus. Stir-fry for about 7 to 10 minutes or until the vegetables are crisp-tender. Add the shrimp and the soy sauce to the pan and stir well. Cook for another 3 minutes or until the shrimp are pink. Add the pineapple and stir to combine. Serve over cooked white or brown rice.

PER SERVING (WITHOUT RICE):

Calories: 240

Total fat: 9 grams

Saturated fat: 1 gram

Cholesterol: 218 milligrams

Sodium: 522 milligrams

Carbohydrate: 15 grams

Dietary fiber: 3 grams

Protein: 26 grams

Calcium: 77 milligrams

Iron: 5 milligrams

Added sugar: 0

MyPlate food groups:

Protein: 4 ounce-equivalents

Vegetable: $3/4$ cup

Fruit: $1/4$ cup

CREAMY POLENTA WITH SAUTEED SHRIMP, SPINACH, AND CHERRY TOMATO BOWL

Makes 2 servings. 🌾

This colorful, satisfying dish includes foods from MyPlate's protein, vegetable, and grain groups.

1/2 cup whole grain cornmeal or dry polenta

1 tablespoon butter

2 tablespoons finely grated Parmesan cheese

1 tablespoon olive oil

1/2 medium onion, peeled and diced

4 cups raw baby spinach, washed and drained, or kale

20 cherry tomatoes, cut in half

3 cloves garlic, peeled and minced

1/4 teaspoon crushed red pepper, if desired

8 ounces large raw shrimp, peeled and cleaned, defrosted if frozen

In a medium saucepan, bring 1 cup of water to a boil. Add the cornmeal, whisking continuously to prevent clumping. Turn heat to low and simmer the cornmeal for 2 to 3 minutes. Add the butter and cheese and continue to whisk for another 2 minutes or until cornmeal achieves a creamy consistency. Remove from heat. Cover and set aside.

In a large skillet, heat the oil over medium heat. Add the onion and sauté for about 3 minutes or until just tender. Add the spinach, tomatoes, and garlic to the pan and sauté, stirring, until the spinach wilts and the tomatoes become tender, about 5 minutes. Add the crushed red pepper and stir. Add the shrimp and cook for about 3 minutes or until the shrimp are pink.

To serve, divide the polenta between two bowls, and top each with half the shrimp-vegetable mixture. Season with fresh ground black pepper, if desired.

PER SERVING:

Calories: 416

Total fat: 17 grams

Saturated fat: 6 grams

Cholesterol: 190 milligrams

Sodium: 340 milligrams

Carbohydrate: 36 grams

Dietary fiber: 9 grams

Protein: 30 grams

Calcium: 200 milligrams

Iron: 6 milligrams

Added sugar: 0

MyPlate food groups:

Protein: 5 ounce-equivalents

Vegetable: $1^1/_2$ cups

Grain: 1 ounce-equivalent
(whole grain)

ROASTED HONEY ORANGE SALMON

Makes 2 servings. (🍾)

Salmon supplies DHA, a beneficial omega-3 fat for baby's brain and vision, and for your well-being. Serve with steamed asparagus or green beans and crusty whole-grain rolls for a balanced meal.

2 tablespoons honey

1/4 cup 100% orange juice

2 tablespoons reduced-sodium soy sauce

2 cloves garlic, peeled and diced, or 1 teaspoon prepared minced garlic

1 tablespoon finely grated, peeled fresh ginger

1/2 teaspoon freshly ground black pepper

8 ounces salmon fillet

Preheat oven to 400°F.

In a small bowl, whisk together the honey, orange juice, soy sauce, garlic, ginger, and black pepper.

Place the salmon skin side down in a shallow baking dish. Top with the honey mixture.

Cook for 15–20 minutes or until the fish flakes easily with a fork.

PER SERVING:

Calories: 333

Total fat: 15 grams

Saturated fat: 3 grams

Cholesterol: 62 milligrams

Sodium: 601 milligrams

Carbohydrate: 25 grams

Dietary fiber: 0

Protein: 24 grams

Calcium: 21 milligrams

Iron: 1 milligram

Added sugar: 17 grams if half of the honey mixture is consumed; about 4 teaspoons

MyPlate food groups:

Protein: 4 ounce-equivalents

BROILED HALIBUT WITH CREAMY DIJON SAUCE

Makes 2 servings.

Halibut harbors a host of nutrients that you and your baby need, including magnesium, iodine, vitamin B6, and potassium.

2 teaspoons butter, melted

4 teaspoons onion powder

$1/_8$ teaspoon dried marjoram

$1/_4$ teaspoon dried thyme, divided

8 ounces halibut filet, about 1-inch thick, skin removed

$1/_4$ cup low-fat sour cream

2 teaspoons all-purpose flour

2 teaspoons Dijon-style mustard

$1/_8$ teaspoon fresh ground black pepper

$1/_2$ cup low-sodium chicken or vegetable broth

Preheat the oven broiler.

In a small bowl, combine the butter, onion powder, marjoram, and $1/_8$ teaspoon thyme. Place the fish on the rack of an unheated broiler pan that's been coated with cooking spray. Brush the fish with the butter mixture. Broil for 5 minutes, turn the fish over, brush with the remaining sauce, and broil for 3 to 7 minutes more, or until the fish flakes easily with a fork.

In a small saucepan, whisk the sour cream with the flour, mustard, black pepper, and remaining $1/_8$ teaspoon thyme. Add the broth, and stir until well mixed. Cook, stirring, over medium heat until the mixture is thickened and bubbly, then cook and stir for 1 minute more. To serve, top the fish with the Dijon sauce.

PER SERVING:

Calories: 257

Total fat: 11 grams

Saturated fat: 5 grams

Cholesterol: 60 milligrams

Sodium: 188 milligrams

Carbohydrate: 11 grams

Dietary fiber: 0

Protein: 28 grams

Calcium: 140 milligrams

Iron: 2 milligrams

Added sugar: 0

MyPlate food groups:

Protein: 4 ounce-equivalents

TURKEY POTPIE

Makes 6 servings.

Nothing says comfort like a potpie. This version is lower in fat and sodium and richer in nutrients than the store-bought kinds.

Filling:

2 cups fresh or frozen chopped carrots

$1/2$ cup low-sodium chicken or vegetable broth or stock

$1^1/2$ cups 1% low-fat milk

$1/3$ cup all-purpose flour

1 teaspoon dried sage leaves, crushed

1 tablespoon butter

$1/2$ teaspoon salt

2 cups cooked turkey (or chicken) breast, cut into $1/2$-inch cubes

1 cup fresh or frozen peas

Topping:

1 cup all-purpose flour

1 teaspoon baking powder

$1/4$ teaspoon salt

$1/8$ teaspoon baking soda

2 tablespoons cold butter, cut into pieces

$1/2$ cup low-fat buttermilk*

Preheat the oven to 400°F. Coat a 2-quart baking dish with cooking spray and set aside.

In a large saucepan, combine the carrots and broth and bring to a boil. Cover and reduce the heat, simmering for 2 to 3 minutes, or until the carrots are crisp-tender.

In a small bowl, whisk together the milk and $1/3$ cup flour and blend well. Stir the milk mixture, sage, butter, and salt into the cooked carrot mixture. Bring to a boil, stirring constantly, then boil for 1 minute longer. Stir in the turkey and peas. Pour the entire filling mixture into the baking dish and set aside while you make the topping.

In a medium bowl, combine the flour, baking powder, salt, and baking soda, and stir. Cut in the butter until the mixture resembles coarse meal. Add the buttermilk, stirring well to mix. Drop by rounded teaspoons onto the turkey mixture, covering it entirely. Bake for 25 to 30 minutes, or until the topping is golden brown.

*You can make buttermilk by pouring 1 tablespoon lemon juice or vinegar into a 1-cup measuring cup. Fill the measuring cup with enough milk to total 1 cup. Let stand for 5 minutes, if possible, then use as you would buttermilk. Save the remaining $1/2$ cup of buttermilk and use in pancakes or quick-bread recipes that call for it.

PER SERVING:

Calories: 298

Total fat: 9 grams

Saturated fat: 5 grams

Cholesterol: 51 milligrams

Sodium: 570 milligrams

Carbohydrate: 33 grams

Dietary fiber: 4 grams

Protein: 22 grams

Calcium: 178 milligrams

Iron: 3 milligrams

Added sugar: 0

MyPlate food groups:

Protein: 4 ounce-equivalents

Vegetable: $1/2$ cup

SHEPHERD'S PIE

Makes 8 servings. (🌾)

A real-crowd pleaser, especially on a chilly day,
and a great way to use up leftover vegetables.

6 medium Yukon Gold potatoes

16 ounces 95% lean ground beef

1 can (10³/₄ ounces) reduced-sodium condensed tomato soup

1 can (14¹/₂ ounces) diced tomatoes with green
pepper, celery, and onion, drained

2 cups green beans, defrosted if frozen

2 cups cooked corn, defrosted if frozen

2 tablespoons trans fat–free tub margarine

1 cup fat-free evaporated milk

1 cup shredded reduced-fat cheddar cheese

Preheat the oven to 350°F. Peel the potatoes and chop into 1-inch
pieces. Place in a medium saucepan and cover with water. Boil over
medium-high heat until fork-tender. Drain potatoes well, return them
to the pan, cover, and set aside.

In a medium skillet coated with cooking spray, brown the meat over
medium-high heat, breaking up the large pieces, until the meat is no
longer pink—about five minutes. Drain well and place in an ungreased
9 x 13–inch baking dish. Add the tomato soup, tomatoes, green beans,
and corn to the meat. Mix well.

Mash the margarine and evaporated milk into the potatoes. Spread the
mashed potatoes evenly on top of the meat and vegetable mixture. Top
with the cheese.

Bake for 20–25 minutes, or until hot. Cool for 5–10 minutes before
serving.

PER SERVING:

Calories: 361

Total fat: 8 grams

Saturated fat: 3 grams

Cholesterol: 47 milligrams

Sodium: 576 milligrams

Carbohydrate: 48 grams

Dietary fiber: 5 grams

Protein: 26 grams

Calcium: 180 milligrams

Iron: 3 milligrams

Added sugar: 0

MyPlate food groups:

Protein: 4 ounce-equivalents

Vegetable: 2 cups

Dairy: $1/2$ cup

TACO SALAD

Makes 1 serving. 🥚 🌾*

*if certified gluten-free oats are used

Black beans and corn lend fiber, phytonutrients, and protein to this nutritious and delicious main dish salad, which is also an excellent source of potassium, folate, and vitamin E.

2 cups romaine lettuce, chopped into 1-inch pieces

1 medium tomato, chopped

$1/4$ avocado, peeled and chopped into 1-inch pieces

$1/2$ cup canned black beans, drained and rinsed well

$1/2$ cup cooked corn, defrosted if frozen

$1/2$ cup crumbled baked tortilla chips

$1/4$ cup shredded reduced-fat Monterey Jack cheese

2 teaspoons canola oil

1 tablespoon fresh lime juice

$1/8$ teaspoon salt

Pinch chili powder (optional)

Pinch ground cumin (optional)

Pinch freshly ground black pepper

Fresh cilantro, chopped (optional)

In a medium bowl, toss together the lettuce, tomato, avocado, beans, and corn. Add the tortilla chips and cheese, and toss a bit more. In a small bowl, whisk together the canola oil, lime juice, salt, chili powder, cumin, and black pepper, and dress the salad. Transfer to a plate. Garnish with cilantro, if desired.

PER SERVING:

Calories: 571

Total fat: 28 grams

Saturated fat: 8 grams

Cholesterol: 28 milligrams

Sodium: 300 milligrams

Carbohydrate: 65 grams

Dietary fiber: 17 grams

Protein: 22 grams

Calcium: 295 milligrams

Iron: 4 milligrams

Added sugar: 0

MyPlate food groups:

Vegetable: 3 cups

Protein: 3 ounce-equivalents

Grain: 1 ounce-equivalent

CHOPPED GREEK SALAD BOWL
Makes 1 serving. 🥗

There are no leafy green vegetables in sight, but this fiber-rich dish is still a salad that can be assembled in about five minutes. Freekeh, a wheat-based whole grain, is typically found in the grain aisle. Use quinoa for a gluten-free salad.

1 tablespoon extra-virgin olive oil

1 tablespoon lemon juice

$1/4$ teaspoon freshly ground black pepper

Pinch dried oregano

1 cup cooked freekeh

$1/4$ cup canned white beans, drained and rinsed

$1/4$ cup chopped peeled cucumber

10 cherry tomatoes, cut in half

5 large olives

2 tablespoons crumbled feta cheese

In a small bowl, whisk together the oil, lemon juice, black pepper, and oregano until well combined. Set aside.

Place the freekeh in a bowl and top with the beans, cucumber, tomatoes, and olives. Top with the dressing and the feta cheese.

PER SERVING:

Calories: 435

Total fat: 23 grams

Saturated fat: 4 grams

Cholesterol: 17 milligrams

Sodium: 695 milligrams

Carbohydrate: 50 grams

Dietary fiber: 12 grams

Protein: 15 grams

Calcium: 186 milligrams

Iron: 7 milligrams

Added sugar: 0

MyPlate food groups:

Protein: 2 ounce-equivalents

Grain: 2 ounce-equivalents
(whole grain)

Vegetable: 1 cup

SANDWICHES, BURGERS, AND PIZZA

BLACK BEAN, CORN, AND CHEESE QUESADILLAS

Makes 2 servings. 🍳

This is so easy yet so good for you, too! Serve with a simple green salad or fruit.

4 7-inch whole-wheat tortillas

$3/4$ cup shredded reduced-fat Monterey Jack cheese

$1/2$ cup cooked black beans, or canned and rinsed

$1/4$ cup corn, defrosted if frozen

2 tablespoons diced red bell pepper

Salsa

Low-fat sour cream

Guacamole

Coat a medium skillet or a griddle with cooking spray or lightly with canola or olive oil. Over low heat, add one of the tortillas (2 if working on a griddle) and top with half of the cheese, beans, corn, and pepper. Cover with another tortilla. Cook for about 2 minutes on each side, gently pressing down on the quesadilla to melt the cheese. Serve with salsa, sour cream, and guacamole, if desired.

PER SERVING (WITHOUT THE SALSA, SOUR CREAM, OR GUACAMOLE):

Calories: 423

Total fat: 6 grams

Saturated fat: 3 grams

Cholesterol: 10 milligrams

Sodium: 919 milligrams

Carbohydrate: 70 grams

Dietary fiber: 12 grams

Protein: 26 grams

Calcium: 230 milligrams

Iron: 4 milligrams

Added sugar: 0 unless the tortillas contain some

MyPlate food groups:

Protein: 4 ounce-equivalents

Grain: 2 ounce-equivalents

Dairy: 1 cup

Vegetable: $1/2$ cup

TUNA BURGERS WITH SMASHED AVOCADO AND TOMATO

Makes 2 servings. (🍼)

These hearty burgers supply omega-3 fats, protein, and many other nutrients you and your baby need. Use salmon in place of tuna, if desired.

2 5¹/₂-ounces cans or pouches of tuna, drained

2 tablespoons seasoned bread crumbs

1 large egg

1 tablespoon finely chopped shallots

1 teaspoon dried dill

2 teaspoons canola oil

¹/₂ pitted avocado, chopped into ¹/₂-inch pieces

1 small tomato, chopped into ¹/₂-inch pieces

2 2-ounce whole-grain sandwich buns or whole-wheat English muffins

Place the tuna in a medium mixing bowl and break it up with a fork. Add the bread crumbs, egg, shallots, and dill, and combine well. Form the mixture into two burgers.

In a medium skillet, heat the oil over medium-high heat. Cook burgers for about 4 minutes on each side.

In a small bowl, combine the avocado and tomato until just mixed, mashing lightly while stirring. To serve, place burgers on sandwich buns and top with the avocado mixture.

PER SERVING:

Calories: 430

Total fat: 14 grams

Saturated fat: 3 grams

Cholesterol: 139 milligrams

Sodium: 810 milligrams

Carbohydrate: 40 grams

Dietary fiber: 8 grams

Protein: 39 grams

Calcium: 108 milligrams

Iron: 4 milligrams

Added sugar: 0 unless the buns or English muffins contain some

MyPlate food groups:

Protein: 6 ounce-equivalents

Grain: 2 ounce-equivalents (whole grain)

GRILLED TURKEY BURGERS WITH WASABI MAYONNAISE

Makes 2 servings.

Cottage cheese boosts the calcium and protein profile and keeps these turkey burgers moist and delicious. You can purchase wasabi paste in a tube at most supermarkets.

$1/4$ cup low-fat cottage cheese

2 teaspoons 1% low-fat milk

8 ounces ground 100% turkey breast

2 teaspoons sesame oil

2 teaspoons reduced-sodium soy sauce

2 cloves garlic, minced

2 scallions, green and white parts, minced

$1/4$ teaspoon freshly ground black pepper

1 large egg

3 tablespoons sesame seeds

1 tablespoon reduced-fat mayonnaise

1 teaspoon wasabi paste

2 2-ounce whole-grain sandwich rolls

Preheat grill to medium-high heat, or heat a large skillet or grill pan that's been coated with cooking spray.

Place the cottage cheese and milk in a blender or food processor and blend until smooth, about 45 seconds.

In a large bowl, combine the cottage cheese mixture with the turkey breast, oil, soy sauce, garlic, scallions, black pepper, egg, and sesame seeds. Mix well. Form into 2 patties.

Grill the burgers until they reach an internal temperature of 165°F as measured by a food thermometer, about 5 to 7 minutes on each side.

In a small bowl, combine the mayonnaise and wasabi paste.

To serve, place the burgers on the buns and top with the wasabi mayonnaise.

PER SERVING:

Calories: 441

Total fat: 19 grams

Saturated fat: 3 grams

Cholesterol: 162 milligrams

Sodium: 517 milligrams

Carbohydrate: 35 grams

Dietary fiber: 6 grams

Protein: 35 grams

Calcium: 249 milligrams

Iron: 5 milligrams

Added sugar: 0, unless the sandwich buns contain some

MyPlate food groups:

Protein: 6 ounce-equivalents

Grain: 2 ounce-equivalents (whole grain)

PORTOBELLO MUSHROOM BURGERS

Makes 2 servings. 🚫

This is a simple, satisfying alternative to beef burgers that won't leave you wanting for meat.

2 large portobello mushroom caps, stems removed, cleaned

1 tablespoon olive oil or canola oil

$1/8$ teaspoon salt

$1/8$ teaspoon freshly ground black pepper

2 1-ounce slices of sharp cheddar cheese

2 2-ounce whole-grain sandwich buns

Sliced tomato and lettuce, if desired

Preheat the oven broiler or grill. Brush the portobello mushroom caps with the oil. Sprinkle with the salt and pepper. Broil or grill the mushrooms until tender, 5 to 10 minutes. Place the cooked mushrooms in buns and top with cheese and lettuce and tomato, if desired.

PER SERVING:

Calories: 279

Total fat: 12 grams

Saturated fat: 3 grams

Cholesterol: 6 milligrams

Sodium: 761 milligrams

Carbohydrate: 33 grams

Dietary fiber: 5 grams

Protein: 14 grams

Calcium: 182 milligrams

Iron: 2 milligrams

Added sugar: 0, unless the sandwich buns contain some

MyPlate food groups:

Grain: 2 ounce-equivalents (whole grain)

Vegetable: 1 cup

Dairy: $1/2$ cup

MEDITERRANEAN WRAP

Makes 1 serving. 🌀

Stock the kitchen with a few prepared foods and you can whip up an interesting and nutritious meal in minutes. Prepared foods, such as hummus, tabouli, and cucumber dip are flavor-filled time-savers.

2-ounce flatbread

1/4 cup prepared hummus

1/2 cup romaine lettuce, shredded

1/4 cup diced tomatoes

2 tablespoons prepared tabouli salad

1/4 cup feta cheese, crumbled

2 tablespoons prepared cucumber dip made with Greek yogurt

Spread the hummus along the middle of the flatbread, leaving about an inch at each end. Layer the lettuce, tomatoes, tabouli, cheese, and cucumber dip on top. Roll flatbread into a wrap. Slice in half to serve.

PER SERVING:

Calories: 504

Total fat: 19 grams

Saturated fat: 4 grams

Cholesterol: 22 milligrams

Sodium: 590 milligrams

Carbohydrate: 50 grams

Dietary fiber: 8 grams

Protein: 15 grams

Calcium: 223 milligrams

Iron: 2 milligrams

Added sugar: 0, unless added to any of the products used

MyPlate food groups:

Grain: 2 ounce-equivalents

Dairy: 3/4 cup

Vegetable: 1/2 cup

RED BELL PEPPER PESTO FLATBREAD

Makes 2 servings. 🚫

Flatbread is used as a thinner pizza crust in this nourishing and delicious dish. You can also swap cooked chopped asparagus or canned, drained quartered artichokes for the peppers.

2 2-ounce pieces of flatbread

1/2 cup part-skim ricotta cheese

3 tablespoons prepared pesto sauce

1/4 cup jarred roasted red peppers, drained and chopped

1/2 cup shredded part-skim mozzarella cheese

Freshly ground black pepper (optional)

Preheat oven to 375° F.

Place the flatbread on a baking sheet. Bake for 4 minutes.

In a small bowl, mix the ricotta cheese and pesto sauce. Spread half the mixture on each flat bread, and top with the red peppers and mozzarella cheese. Season with black pepper, if desired. Bake for 5 minutes.

PER SERVING:

Calories: 472

Total fat: 23 grams

Saturated fat: 7 grams

Cholesterol: 23 milligrams

Sodium: 925 milligrams

Carbohydrate: 45 grams

Dietary fiber: 7 grams

Protein: 25 grams

Calcium: 390 milligrams

Iron: 3 milligrams

Added sugar: 0

MyPlate food groups:

Grain: 1 ounce-equivalent

Dairy: 1/2 cup

TOMATO, ARUGULA, AND FETA CHEESE PIZZA

Makes 4 servings. 🚫

*Arugula's slightly peppery taste adds some
depth to this pizza, which is part salad.*

10-ounce prepared whole-wheat thin pizza crust

2 medium tomatoes, sliced

$1/3$ cup grated Parmesan cheese

2 cups arugula

1 tablespoon olive oil

2 teaspoons lemon juice

$1/2$ cup crumbled feta cheese

Preheat oven to 400°F.

Place the pizza crust on a baking sheet. Top with tomato slices and sprinkle with Parmesan cheese. Bake for 10 minutes.

In a medium bowl, toss the arugula with the oil and lemon juice. Top the warm pizza crust with the arugula mixture, spreading evenly. Sprinkle feta cheese on top.

Return to the oven and bake for 5 minutes. Serve warm.

PER SERVING ($1/4$ OF THE PIZZA):

Calories: 308

Total fat: 14 grams

Saturated fat: 6 grams

Cholesterol: 24 milligrams

Sodium: 686 milligrams

Carbohydrate: 37 grams

Dietary fiber: 7 grams

Protein: 14 grams

Calcium: 266 milligrams

Iron: 1 milligram

Added sugar: 0, unless there is sugar in the pizza crust

MyPlate food groups:

Grain: 2 ounce-equivalents

Vegetable: $3/4$ cup

Dairy: $1/4$ cup

CAULIFLOWER CRUST PERSONAL PIZZA WITH MUSHROOMS, OLIVES, AND GOAT CHEESE

Makes 4 servings. 🍽 🌾

Ricing cauliflower is easy, but you can skip a step by using the prepared variety. Mix up the vegetable toppings to your liking on this gluten-free crust.

2 cups riced cauliflower*

$1/2$ cup shredded part-skim mozzarella cheese

2 large eggs

1 teaspoon dried oregano

$1/4$ teaspoon salt

$1/4$ teaspoon freshly ground black pepper

2 teaspoons olive oil

8 ounces sliced white button or baby bella mushrooms

10 medium pitted Kalamata olives, chopped

4 ounces goat cheese, crumbled

Preheat oven to 425°F. Line a large baking sheet with parchment paper and coat with cooking spray.

In a large bowl, stir together the cauliflower, mozzarella cheese, eggs, oregano, salt, and black pepper. Spoon the cauliflower mixture into 4 circles on the baking sheet, and shape each one into a 4-inch, flat round, pressing the ingredients together with your hands or the back of a spoon. Bake for 15 minutes, then flip and bake for another 10 minutes.

Heat oil in a large skillet over medium heat. Add the mushrooms and sauté until tender, about 10 minutes. Drain.

In a medium bowl, combine the mushrooms, olives, and goat cheese. Spread the toppings on each crust, and return to the oven to bake for another 5 minutes.

*To rice cauliflower, remove the stems and leaves from the head, and chop the florets into large chunks. Place in a food processer and pulse until the cauliflower looks like grain, about 10 times. You can also use a cheese grater to make riced cauliflower. A large head of cauliflower produces about 3 cups riced cauliflower. Use leftover riced cauliflower in salads, soups, and add to mac and cheese recipes, or freeze for later use. Riced cauliflower is also available in the frozen foods aisle.

PER SERVING:

Calories: 271

Total fat: 18 grams

Saturated fat: 9 grams

Cholesterol: 135 milligrams

Sodium: 635 milligrams

Carbohydrate: 14 grams

Dietary fiber: 5 grams

Protein: 18 grams

Calcium: 259 milligrams

Iron: 3 milligrams

Added sugar: 0

MyPlate food groups:

Protein: 2 ounce-equivalents

Vegetable: $3/4$ cup

Dairy: $3/4$ cup

BROCCOLI CHEESE CALZONE
Makes 8 servings. 🥄

You're four ingredients away from a calzone that beats pizza shop versions in both nutritional value and taste.

3 teaspoons olive oil, divided

10 cups chopped broccoli florets

16 ounces prepared pizza dough

16-ounce block (or 2 8-ounce blocks) cheddar cheese

Preheat oven to 400°F. Lightly coat a large baking sheet with 1 teaspoon of the oil.

Steam the broccoli. When the broccoli is fork-tender, rinse with cool water. Drain well and blot with a clean towel to remove excess moisture.

Slice the cheddar cheese into $1/4$-inch slices. (You can substitute packaged shredded cheese.)

On a lightly floured surface, roll out the pizza dough into a rectangle about 10 inches long and 16 inches wide. Sprinkle half the cheese on half of the pizza dough to within $1/2$ inch of the edge of the dough.

Arrange the broccoli evenly over the cheese. Cover the broccoli with the remaining cheese. Fold the dough over the broccoli and cheese filling, and seal the edges with the tines of a fork.

Carefully transfer the calzone to the baking sheet. Brush the calzone with the remaining oil.

Cook for about 20 minutes, or until the crust is golden brown. Allow the calzone to rest for at least 5 minutes before cutting.

Warm leftovers for about 7 minutes in a 300°F oven, or for about 30 seconds in the microwave.

PER SERVING:

Calories: 270

Total fat: 8 grams

Saturated fat: 3 grams

Cholesterol: 12 milligrams

Sodium: 820 milligrams

Carbohydrate: 33 grams

Dietary fiber: 5 grams

Protein: 22 grams

Calcium: 286 milligrams

Iron: 1 milligram

Added sugar: 0

MyPlate food groups:

Grain: 2 ounce-equivalents

Dairy: 1 cup

SOUPS AND STEWS

CHICKEN AND WHITE BEAN CHILI
Makes 8 servings. 🌾

Beans are bursting with protein, fiber, and antioxidants that protect your cells—and your baby's. Make a batch of this chili and freeze the leftovers.

1 tablespoon olive oil

2 medium onions, peeled and chopped

3 cloves garlic, peeled and minced

4 cups canned great northern beans, drained and rinsed well

4 cups low-sodium chicken or vegetable broth

3 cups cooked, cubed skinless chicken breast, cut into $1/2$-inch cubes

2 teaspoons ground cumin

$1/2$ teaspoon ground cloves

1 teaspoon dried oregano

2 cups (8 ounces) shredded Monterey Jack Cheese

In a large saucepan, heat the oil over medium heat. Add the onions and sauté until they are nearly clear, about 4 to 5 minutes. Add the garlic and sauté for another minute. Add the beans, broth, chicken, cumin, cloves, and oregano to the pan. Turn heat to low. Cover the saucepan and simmer for about 1 hour. Before serving, remove from the heat and stir in the cheese until it melts.

PER SERVING:

Calories: 387

Total fat: 13 grams

Saturated fat: 6 grams

Cholesterol: 70 milligrams

Sodium: 233 milligrams

Carbohydrate: 32 grams

Dietary fiber: 7 grams

Protein: 36 grams

Calcium: 299 milligrams

Iron: 3 milligrams

Added sugar: 0

MyPlate food groups:

Protein: 5 ounce-equivalents

Dairy: 1 cup

Vegetables: 1 cup

CREAMY SWEET POTATO SOUP

Makes 4 servings. 🍖* 🌾

*if vegetable broth is used

*Short on time? Substitute canned sweet potato
for this potassium- and calcium-packed soup.
Use vegetable broth and soy milk to make it vegan.*

1 tablespoon canola oil

1 medium onion, peeled and diced

4 medium sweet potatoes, cooked, peeled, and chopped into 2-inch cubes

1 cup low-sodium chicken broth or vegetable broth

$1/4$ teaspoon ground ginger

$1/4$ teaspoon ground cumin

2 cups 2% reduced-fat milk, or unsweetened fortified soy milk

In a medium saucepan, heat the oil over medium heat. Add the onions and sauté until nearly clear, about 4 to 5 minutes. Transfer the onions to a blender or a food processor. Add the sweet potatoes, chicken broth or stock, ginger, and cumin. Puree until smooth. Return the mixture to the saucepan and add the milk. Warm gently. Serve immediately.

Note: Don't add the milk to the vegetable mixture if you don't plan to eat all of the soup immediately. Take what you plan to eat of the sweet potato puree and add enough milk to achieve the desired consistency. Freeze the remaining sweet potato mixture, or store it covered tightly in the refrigerator for up to 3 days. Add the milk as you use the puree.

PER SERVING:

Calories: 203

Total fat: 6 grams

Saturated fat: 2 grams

Cholesterol: 10 milligrams

Sodium: 105 milligrams

Carbohydrate: 30 grams

Dietary fiber: 4 grams

Protein: 8 grams

Calcium: 189 milligrams

Iron: 1 milligram

Added sugar: 0

MyPlate food groups:

Vegetable: 1 cup

Dairy: $1/2$ cup

VEGGIE "STOUP"

Makes 6 servings.

This dish is not quite a soup, and not quite
a stew, but quite delicious and nutritious!
Enjoy some now, and save the rest for later.

2 tablespoons olive oil

$1/2$ cup diced carrots

3 stalks celery, diced

2 medium onions, peeled and diced

6 cloves garlic, minced

4 cups chopped zucchini

1 cup peeled, cubed eggplant

1 cup low-sodium vegetable broth or stock

1 can (28-ounce) no-salt-added diced tomatoes, undrained

2 cups chopped raw kale

1 can (19-ounce) garbanzo beans, drained

2 teaspoons dried parsley

1 teaspoon dried thyme

1 teaspoon dried rosemary

1 teaspoon salt

$1/2$ teaspoon freshly ground black pepper

In a large saucepan, heat the oil over medium-high heat. Add the carrots, celery, onions, and garlic. Cook the vegetables until the onions are nearly clear, about 4 to 5 minutes. Add the zucchini and eggplant and cook for 5 to 7 minutes. Add the broth or stock and continue to cook for another 5 minutes. Add the tomatoes and their juice, kale, and beans. Bring the mixture to a boil. Season with the parsley, thyme, rosemary, salt, and pepper. Add more broth for a thinner consistency.

Serve over cooked quinoa, freekeh, or farro for additional protein, fiber, and whole grains.

PER SERVING (WITHOUT ADDED GRAINS):

Calories: 213

Total fat: 6 grams

Saturated fat: 1 gram

Cholesterol: 0

Sodium: 307 milligrams

Carbohydrate: 35 grams

Dietary fiber: 8 grams

Protein: 8 grams

Calcium: 131 milligrams

Iron: 3 milligrams

Added sugar: 0

MyPlate food groups:

Vegetables: 2 cups

Protein: 1 ounce-equivalent

SLOW-COOKER BEEF AND MUSHROOM STEW
Makes 6 servings. (🥃)

Mushrooms have umami, a taste sensation that brings a savory flavor to dishes. Vary this stew with a mixture of mushrooms, such as white button and shiitake.

1 medium onion, chopped

2 cups baby carrots

16 ounces sliced baby bella mushrooms

1 can (15-ounce) no-salt-added diced tomatoes, undrained

$1^1/_2$ cups reduced-sodium beef broth

$^1/_2$ cup all-purpose flour

1 teaspoon salt

1 teaspoon dried marjoram

1 pound stew meat, such as chuck, cut into $^1/_2$-inch pieces

1 cup fresh or frozen peas

Freshly ground black pepper to taste (optional)

Place all the ingredients except the beef, peas, and pepper in a slow cooker. Combine well. Add the beef. Cover and cook on the low setting for 8 hours. Just before serving, add the peas and season with pepper, if desired. Stir well. Cover and cook for 5 more minutes.

PER SERVING:

Calories: 238

Total fat: 5 grams

Saturated fat: 2 grams

Cholesterol: 54 milligrams

Sodium: 470 milligrams

Carbohydrate: 22 grams

Dietary fiber: 4 grams

Protein: 27 grams

Calcium: 39 milligrams

Iron: 3 milligrams

Added sugar: 0

MyPlate food groups:

Protein: 4 ounce-equivalents

Vegetable: 1 cup

VEGETABLES AND SIDE DISHES

MASHED POTATOES WITH GREENS AND CHEESE

Makes 4 servings. 🖤 🌾

Evaporated milk supplies twice the calcium of regular milk, which gives a serving of this side dish as much calcium as a glass of milk. You can use plain yogurt in place of sour cream.

4 medium Yukon Gold potatoes, washed and quartered

$1/2$ cup fat-free evaporated milk

2 tablespoons low-fat sour cream

$3/4$ cup shredded Gouda or fontina cheese

2 cups chopped raw collard greens

Freshly ground black pepper, if desired

In a medium saucepan, boil the potatoes for about 15 to 20 minutes or until tender. Drain well and return to the pan. Add the milk and the sour cream and mash into the potatoes. Transfer the mixture to a serving bowl. Add the cheese and collard greens, and mix well. Serve warm.

PER SERVING:

Calories: 246

Total fat: 7 grams

Saturated fat: 4 grams

Cholesterol: 27 milligrams

Sodium: 228 milligrams

Carbohydrate: 34 grams

Dietary fiber: 5 grams

Protein: 12 grams

Calcium: 300 milligrams

Iron: 1 milligram

Added sugar: 0

MyPlate food groups:

Vegetable: 2 cups

Dairy: $1/2$ cup

QUINOA SALAD WITH TOASTED PECANS AND DRIED APRICOTS

Makes 6 servings. 🌾 🍾

Quinoa, a naturally gluten-free grain, is easy to cook and is a higher-protein alternative to regular pasta and white rice.

2 cups low-sodium chicken or vegetable broth or stock

1 cup quinoa, uncooked

$1/2$ cup dried apricots with no added sugar, chopped into $1/4$-inch pieces, or golden raisins

$1/2$ cup chopped pecans, toasted*

$1/4$ cup sliced scallions

3 tablespoons olive oil

3 tablespoons balsamic vinegar

In a medium saucepan, bring the broth to a boil over high heat. Add the quinoa to the pan and cover. Reduce the heat to low and allow quinoa to simmer for about 20 minutes, or until the broth is absorbed. Uncover, stir, and allow to cool for 15 minutes.

In a medium bowl, combine the apricots, pecans, and scallions. Set aside.

In a small bowl, make the dressing by whisking the oil and vinegar together until well blended. When the quinoa is cool, add the apricot-nut mixture and dressing to the pan, and stir to combine well. Transfer to a serving bowl. Cover and chill for about 30 minutes before eating, or serve immediately.

*Toasting pecans makes them even more flavorful. Preheat oven to 300°F. Spread the pecan pieces in a single layer on a nonstick baking sheet. Cook for about 10 minutes or until the nuts turn slightly darker, turning them with a spatula halfway through. Cool before chopping.

PER SERVING:

Calories: 266

Total fat: 16 grams

Saturated fat: 2 grams

Cholesterol: 0

Sodium: 27 milligrams

Carbohydrate: 27 grams

Dietary fiber: 4 grams

Protein: 7 grams

Calcium: 29 milligrams

Iron: 2 milligrams

Added sugar: 0

MyPlate food groups:

Grain: $1^1/_2$ ounce-equivalents
(whole grain)

FARRO WITH BEETS, PISTACHIOS, AND FETA CHEESE
Makes 4 servings. (🚫)

Farro is an ancient grain rich in protein and fiber, and it supplies iron. Use packaged precooked beets for convenience.

1 cup pearled farro

2 tablespoons plus 1 teaspoon fresh lemon juice

1 tablespoon olive oil

$1/2$ teaspoon salt

$1/2$ teaspoon freshly ground black pepper

1 cup cooked, peeled beets (2 medium), chopped into $1/4$-inch pieces

$1/4$ cup feta cheese, crumbled

$1/4$ cup chopped shelled pistachios

In a medium saucepan, bring 2 cups water to a boil. Add the farro to the pan and cover. Reduce the heat to low and allow farro to simmer for 20 to 25 minutes, or until the water is absorbed.

In a small bowl, make the dressing by whisking the lemon juice, oil, salt, and black pepper together until well blended.

Place the farro in a serving bowl. Add the dressing and mix well. Top with the beets, feta cheese, and pistachios and serve.

PER SERVING:

Calories: 290

Total fat: 10 grams

Saturated fat: 2 grams

Cholesterol: 8 milligrams

Sodium: 435 milligrams

Carbohydrate: 42 grams

Dietary fiber: 7 grams

Protein: 11 grams

Calcium: 80 milligrams

Iron: 3 milligrams

Added sugar: 0

MyPlate food groups:

Grain: 2 ounce-equivalents (whole grain)

ROASTED VEGETABLE MEDLEY

Makes 4 servings. 🥩 🌾 🍼

Roasting brings out the natural flavors in vegetables. You can roast nearly any vegetable, so use your imagination to vary this side dish, which pairs well with meat, chicken, and fish.

1 pound red-skinned potatoes (about 10 small), washed and quartered

1 cup cubed raw carrots (1-inch cubes)

1 cup raw broccoli florets

1 cup raw cauliflower florets

2 small onions, peeled and cut into 4 wedges each

1/4 cup olive oil

3 cloves garlic, peeled and minced

1 teaspoon dried rosemary

1 teaspoon dried basil

Salt (optional)

Preheat the oven to 400°F. Place the vegetables in a large mixing bowl and set aside.

In a small bowl, make the dressing by whisking together the oil, garlic, rosemary, and basil until well blended. Drizzle the mixture over the vegetables and stir well to fully coat. Spread the vegetable combination on an ungreased 9 x 13–inch baking sheet. Roast for about 20 minutes, or until the vegetables become fork-tender; toss after 10 minutes in the oven. Season with salt, if desired.

PER SERVING (WITHOUT SALT):

Calories: 243

Total fat: 14 grams

Saturated fat: 2 grams

Cholesterol: 0

Sodium: 45 milligrams

Carbohydrate: 27 grams

Dietary fiber: 5 grams

Protein: 4 grams

Calcium: 50 milligrams

Iron: 1 milligram

Added sugar: 0

MyPlate food groups:

Vegetable: 1 1/2 cups

CAULIFLOWER STEAKS WITH LEMON TAHINI SAUCE

Makes 3 servings. 🥩 🌾 🫒

Tahini, made from ground sesame seeds,
is loaded with heart-healthy fats.

1 large head cauliflower

2 tablespoons olive oil

1/4 cup tahini

1 clove garlic, peeled and minced, or 1/2 teaspoon prepared minced garlic

5 tablespoons fresh lemon juice

1/4 teaspoon salt

Pinch ground cumin, if desired

Preheat the oven to 400°F.

Trim the leaves and the root end off the cauliflower and slice into 2-inch-thick slabs. Brush each side of the cauliflower and the florets with the oil. Place on a baking sheet, and roast until tender, about 18–20 minutes.

To make the dressing, place the tahini, garlic, lemon juice, salt, and cumin in a blender or food processor. Blend until smooth, about 45 seconds to 1 minute.

To serve, drizzle the tahini sauce on the warm cauliflower.

PER SERVING:

Calories: 229

Total fat: 16 grams

Saturated fat: 2 grams

Cholesterol: 0

Sodium: 301 milligrams

Carbohydrate: 19 grams

Dietary fiber: 9 grams

Protein: 9 grams

Calcium: 147 milligrams

Iron: 3 milligrams

Added sugar: 0

MyPlate food groups:

Vegetable: 1 cup

DESSERTS AND SNACKS

CHOCOLATE AVOCADO PUDDING

Makes 2 servings. 🔘 🌾 🍾

This rich and creamy plant-based pudding only feels like a splurge! It's packed with healthy fats, phytonutrients, and fiber.

1 ripe banana, broken into large chunks

1 ripe avocado, pitted, peeled, and cut into large chunks

2 tablespoons unsweetened cocoa powder

1 tablespoon pure maple syrup

Place the banana, avocado, cocoa powder, and maple syrup in a food processor. Process until smooth, about 45 seconds to 1 minute. Divide into two bowls and serve.

PER SERVING:

Calories: 251

Total fat: 16 grams

Saturated fat: 3 grams

Cholesterol: 0

Sodium: 10 milligrams

Carbohydrate: 32 grams

Dietary fiber: 10 grams

Protein: 4 grams

Calcium: 28 milligrams

Iron: 2 milligrams

Added sugar: 7 grams; about 2 teaspoons

MyPlate food groups:

Fruit: 1 cup

DATE NUT BALLS

Makes 26 balls. 🥜 🌾 🍶

*You can make these portable goodies in a snap. Take
them with you for when hunger strikes between meals!*

2 cups dry-roasted peanuts or roasted almonds

24 whole pitted dates, roughly chopped

$1/4$ cup unsweetened cocoa powder

2 tablespoons natural crunchy peanut butter

1 teaspoon pure vanilla extract

Place the peanuts or almonds in a food processor and process until
crumbly. Remove the nuts from the food processor and place in a small
bowl. Add the dates to the food processor and process until they become
sticky. Add back the nuts to the food processor, and add the cocoa
powder, peanut butter, and vanilla extract. Pulse until all the ingredients
are mixed together, scraping down the bowl to combine well. Form into
26 balls.

Store in an airtight container. Refrigerate or freeze.

PER SERVING (2 BALLS):

Calories: 179

Total fat: 12 grams

Saturated fat: 2 grams

Cholesterol: 0

Sodium: 191 milligrams

Carbohydrate: 15 grams

Dietary fiber: 3 grams

Protein: 6 grams

Calcium: 18 milligrams

Iron: 1 milligram

Added sugar: 0, unless there is some
in the peanut butter.

MyPlate food groups:

Protein: 1 ounce-equivalent

BLACK BEAN BROWNIE BITES

Makes 24 brownies.

*Nobody has to know about the black
beans in these fudgy mini treats!*

1 15-ounce can black beans,
rinsed and drained

1/4 cup canola oil

2 large eggs

3/4 cup granulated sugar

1/2 cup unsweetened cocoa
powder

1 teaspoon pure vanilla extract

1/2 teaspoon baking powder

1/2 teaspoon salt

2/3 cup semisweet chocolate
mini baking chips

Preheat oven to 350°F. Coat a 24-muffin pan with cooking spray.

Place the beans and the oil in a food processor. Process on high until
smooth, about 2 to 3 minutes. Add the eggs, sugar, cocoa powder, and
vanilla extract and blend well. Add the baking powder and salt and blend
for 10 seconds more. Stir in the baking chips.

Pour the batter by rounded tablespoons into each muffin cup. Bake for
10 minutes or until a toothpick inserted in the middle of a brownie bite
comes out clean. Cool on a wire rack for 5 minutes, then remove from
the pan and cool completely.

PER SERVING (1 BROWNIE BITE):

Calories: 102 calories

Total fat: 5 grams

Saturated fat: 1 gram

Cholesterol: 18 milligrams

Sodium: 42 milligrams

Carbohydrate: 14 grams

Dietary fiber: 2 grams

Protein: 2 grams

Calcium: 15 milligrams

Iron: 1 milligram

Added sugar: 11 grams; about 3
teaspoons

MyPlate food groups:

None

CHOCOLATE RAISIN CLUSTERS
Makes 8 servings. 🦐 🌾

*Craving candy? These fruit and chocolate
goodies will hit the spot. Use unsweetened dried
cherries in place of raisins if you'd like.*

6 ounces bittersweet chocolate chips

1 cup raisins

Melt the chocolate in the top of a double boiler, stirring constantly, or
melt in a large glass bowl in the microwave according to package directions.
When the chocolate has melted, remove the top portion of the
double boiler and turn off the burner. Add the raisins to the chocolate
and stir, completely coating the fruit. Drop the chocolate-raisin mixture
by heaping teaspoons onto wax paper to form 16 clusters. Allow to cool
completely.

PER SERVING (2 CLUSTERS):

Calories: 170 calories

Total fat: 6 grams

Saturated fat: 3 grams

Cholesterol: 1 milligram

Sodium: 3 milligrams

Carbohydrate: 30 grams

Dietary fiber: 2 grams

Protein: 2 grams

Calcium: 18 milligrams

Iron: 1 milligram

Added sugar: 11 grams; about
3 teaspoons (from the chocolate)

MyPlate food groups:

None

NO-COOK NUT BUTTER CRUNCHIES

Makes 8 servings. 🥜 🌾

A cross between candy and cookie, these sweet and crunchy delights serve up heart-healthy fat, protein, and calcium.

$1/2$ cup natural smooth almond, peanut, soy-nut, or sunflower seed butter

$1/2$ cup honey

1 teaspoon pure vanilla extract

$3/4$ cup powdered nonfat milk

$2/3$ cup crispy rice cereal

In a large bowl, blend the almond (or other) butter, honey, and vanilla extract. Add the powdered milk and cereal. Mix well and form into 16 balls.

PER SERVING (2 CRUNCHIES):

Calories: 191

Total fat: 8 grams

Saturated fat: 2 grams

Cholesterol: 1 milligram

Sodium: 131 milligrams

Carbohydrate: 26 grams

Dietary fiber: 1 gram

Protein: 7 grams

Calcium: 87 milligrams

Iron: 1 milligram

Added sugar: 17 grams; about 4 teaspoons

MyPlate food groups:

Protein: 1 ounce-equivalent

Dairy: $1/3$ cup

STRAWBERRY CHIA PUDDING

Makes 2 servings. 🌀 🌾

Kefir is similar to drinkable yogurt in consistency, but usually contains more live active cultures to help keep you regular and support your immune system. Look for kefir in the dairy case.

1 cup fresh or frozen whole strawberries

1 tablespoon honey (more if desired)

1 cup plain kefir

$^1/_2$ cup 1% low-fat milk

5 tablespoons chia seeds

Place the strawberries, honey, and kefir in a blender or food processor and blend on high until smooth, about 2 minutes.

In a medium bowl, combine the milk and chia seeds. Add the strawberry mixture and stir to combine. Cover and refrigerate for at least 8 hours before eating.

PER SERVING:

Calories: 248

Total fat: 11 grams

Saturated fat: 3 grams

Cholesterol: 18 milligrams

Sodium: 94 milligrams

Carbohydrate: 32 grams

Dietary fiber: 9 grams

Protein: 10 grams

Calcium: 353 milligrams

Iron: 0

Added sugar: 9 grams; about 2 teaspoons

MyPlate food groups:

Dairy: 1 cup

Fruit: $^1/_2$ cup

MANGO ICE "MILK"

Makes 2 servings. 🍥 🌾 🍾

This creamy treat is dairy-free! If you freeze the fruit in advance, this dessert can be ready in less than five minutes.

1 cup chopped frozen mango

1 frozen banana, peeled and sliced (peel and slice before freezing)

$1/3$ cup reduced-fat coconut milk

2 teaspoons lime juice

Place the mango, banana, coconut milk, and lime juice in a food processor. Process on high until creamy, about 1 minute.

Top with chia seeds, flaked coconut, or chopped pistachios, if desired.

PER SERVING (WITHOUT TOPPINGS):

Calories: 139

Total fat: 3 grams

Saturated fat: 3 grams

Cholesterol: 0

Sodium: 12 milligrams

Carbohydrate: 29 grams

Dietary fiber: 3 grams

Protein: 2 grams

Calcium: 11 milligrams

Iron: 0

Added sugar: 0

MyPlate food groups:

Fruit: 1 cup

References

1. PREPREGNANCY: STARTING FROM A HEALTHY PLACE

Academy of Nutrition and Dietetics. "Position of the Academy of Nutrition and Dietetics: Nutrition and Lifestyle for a Healthy Pregnancy Outcome." *Journal of the Academy of Nutrition and Dietetics* 114:1099–1103, 2014.

Allen, L. "Multiple Micronutrients in Pregnancy and Lactation: An Overview." *American Journal of Clinical Nutrition* 81:1206S–1212S, 2005.

American Academy of Pediatrics. "Clinical Report: Fetal Alcohol Spectrum Disorders." Year. 2015,http://pediatrics.aappublications.org/content/pediatrics/early/2015/10/13/peds.2015-3113.full.pdf.

American Academy of Pediatrics and the American College of Obstetricians and Gynecologists. *Guidelines for Perinatal Care,* 7th ed. Elk Grove Village, IL: AAP and ACOG, 2012.

American College of Obstetricians and Gynecologists. "Committee Opinion: Moderate Caffeine Consumption During Pregnancy." 2010. www.acog.org/-/media/Committee-Opinions/Committee-on-Obstetric-Practice/co462.pdf?dmc=1&ts=20160124T1428453501.

———. "Committee Opinion: Oral Health Care During Pregnancy and Through the Lifespan." 2015. www.acog.org/Resources-And-Publications/Committee-Opinions/Committee-on-Health-Care-for-Underserved-Women/Oral-Health-Care-During-Pregnancy-and-Through-the-Lifespan#20.

———. "Good Health Before Pregnancy: Preconception Care." 2015. www.acog.org/Patients/FAQs/Good-Health-Before-Pregnancy-Preconception-Care.

American Society for Reproductive Medicine. "Infertility: An Overview." 2012. www.asrm.org/Booklet_Infertility_An_Overview.

————. "Optimizing Natural Fertility." 2015. www.reproductivefacts.org/uploadedFiles/ASRM_Content/Resources/Patient_Resources/Fact_Sheets_and_Info_Booklets/Optimizing%20natural%20fertility%204-23-12%20FINAL.pdf.

————. "Quick Facts About Fertility." www.asrm.org/detail.aspx?id=2322.

American Thyroid Association. "Hypothryroidism." 2014. http://www.thyroid.org/wp-content/uploads/patients/brochures/Hypo_brochure.pdf

Bailey, B., and Sokol, R. "Prenatal Alcohol Exposure and Miscarriage, Stillbirth, Preterm Delivery, and Sudden Infant Death Syndrome." *Alcohol Research & Health* 34:86–91, 2011.

Bailey, L., and Berry, R. "Folic Acid Supplementation and the Occurrence of Congenital Heart Defects, Orofacial Clefts, Multiple Births, and Miscarriage." *American Journal of Clinical Nutrition* 81:1213S–1217S, 2005.

Bergholt, T., et al. "Maternal Body Mass Index in the First Trimester and Risk of Cesarean Delivery in Nulliparous Women in Spontaneous Labor." *American Journal of Obstetrics and Gynecology* 96:163e1–163e5, 2007.

Berry, R., et al. "Prevention of Neural Tube Defects with Folic Acid in China." *New England Journal of Medicine* 341:1485–1490, 1999.

Botto, L., et al. "Occurrence of Congenital Heart Defects in Relation to Maternal Mulitivitamin Use." *American Journal of Epidemiology* 151:878–884, 2000.

Buck Louis, G., et al. "Lifestyle and Pregnancy Loss in a Contemporary Cohort of Women Recruited Before Conception: The LIFE Study." *Fertility and Sterility* 106:180–188, 2016.

Catov, J., et al. "Periconceptual Multivitamin Use and Risk of Preterm or Small-for-Gestational Age Births in the Danish National Birth Cohort." *American Journal of Clinical Nutrition* 93:906–912, 2011.

Centers for Disease Control and Prevention. "About Prediabetes and Type 2 Diabetes." 2016. www.cdc.gov/diabetes/prevention/prediabetes-type2/index.html.

————. "Folic Acid: Questions and Answers." 2015. www.cdc.gov/ncbddd/folicacid/faqs.html

————. "Infertility FAQs. What Is Infertility?" 2016.www.cdc.gov/reproductivehealth/infertility.

————. "Folic Acid Recommendations." 2016. www.cdc.gov/ncbddd/folic acid/recommenations.html.

————. "National Diabetes Statistics Report, 2014." 2014. www.cdc.gov/diabetes/pubs/statsreport14/national-diabetes-report-web.pdf.

————. "Preconception Health and Health Care." 2016. www.cdc.gov/preconception/index.html.

————. "Tobacco Use and Pregnancy: How Does Smoking During Pregnancy Harm

My Health and My Baby?" 2016. www.cdc.gov/reproductivehealth/maternalinfanthealth/
tobaccousepregnancy/index.htm.

———. "Vaccines Schedules." 2016. http://www.cdc.gov/vaccines/schedules/index.html

———. "What You Should Know About Alcohol and Pregnancy." 2014. www.cdc.gov/
features/alcoholandpregnancy/.

Chang, J., and Servey, J. "Over-the-Counter Medications in Pregnancy." *American Family Physician* 90:548–555, 2014.

Chavarro, J., et al. "Diet and Lifestyle in the Prevention of Ovulatory Disorder Infertility." *Obstetrics and Gynecology* 110:1050–1058, 2007.

Cleveland Clinic. "Drugs and Male Fertility." 2013. https://my.clevelandclinic.org/health/
diseases_conditions/hic-advanced-semen-tests-for-fertility/hic-drugs-and-male-fertility.

Czeizel, A. "The Primary Prevention of Birth Defects: Multivitamins or Folic Acid?" *International Journal of Medical Sciences* 1:50–61, 2004.

Dante G., et al. "Herb Remedies During Pregnancy." *Journal of Maternal and Fetal Neonatal Medicine* 26:306–312, 2013.

Dean, S., et al. "Born Too Soon: Care Before and Between Pregnancy to Prevent Preterm Births: From Evidence to Action." *Reproductive Health* 10:S3, 2013.

Food and Drug Administration. "Tips for Dietary Supplement Users." 2014. www.fda.
gov/Food/DietarySupplements/UsingDietarySupplements/ucm110567.htm.

Gensink Law, D. "Obesity and Time to Pregnancy." *Human Reproduction* 22:414–420, 2007.

Goh, Y. I., et al. "Prenatal Multivitamin Supplementation and Rates of Congenital Anomalies: A Meta-Analysis." *Journal of Obstetrics and Gynaecology of Canada* 28:680–689, 2006.

Hyland, A., et al. "Associations Between Lifetime Tobacco Exposure with Infertility and Age at Natural Menopause: The Women's Health Initiative Observational Study. Tobacco Control." Published online first: 14 December 2015. doi:10.1136/tobaccocontrol-2015-052510.

Kesmodel, U., et al. "Moderate Alcohol Intake During Pregnancy and the Risk of Stillbirth and Death in the First Year of Life." *American Journal of Epidemiology* 155:305–312, 2002.

Klonoff-Cohen, H., et al. "A Prospective Study of the Effects of Female and Male Caffeine Consumption on the Reproductive Endpoints of IVG and Gamete Intra-Fallopian Transfer." *Human Reproduction* 17:1746–1754. 2002.

March of Dimes. "Caffeine in Pregnancy." 2015. www.marchofdimes.org/pregnancy/
caffeine-in-pregnancy.aspx.

———. "Electronic Cigarettes and Pregnancy." 2015. www.marchofdimes.org/materials/e-Cigarettes-and-Pregnancy-Fact-Sheet-March-2015.pdf.

———. "Secondhand Smoke and Your Baby." 2014. www.marchofdimes.org/secondhand-smoke-and-your-baby.aspx.

———. "Your Check-Up Before Pregnancy." 2013. www.marchofdimes.org/pregnancy/your-checkup-before-pregnancy.aspx.

Mayo Clinic. "Celiac Disease." 2016. http://www.mayoclinic.org/diseases-conditions/celiac-disease/home/ovc-

———. "Male Infertility." 2015. www.mayoclinic.org/diseases-conditions/male-infertility/basics/causes/CON-20033113.

Mostafa, T. "Cigarette Smoking and Male Fertility." *Journal of Advanced Research* 1:179–186, 2010.

National Academies of Science, Institute of Medicine. *Weight Gain During Pregnancy: Reexamining the Guidelines.* Washington, DC: National Academies Press, 2009.

National Diabetes Education Initiative. "Diabetes Management Guidelines: American Diabetes Association (ADA) 2015 Guidelines." www.ndei.org/ADA-diabetes-management-guidelines-diabetes-in-pregnancy-GDM.aspx.

National Institute of Diabetes and Digestive and Kidney Diseases. "Celiac Disease and Reproductive Problems." www.celiac.nih.gov/ReproductiveProblems.aspx.

———. "Do You Know Some of the Health Risks of Being Overweight?" 2012. http://www.niddk.nih.gov/health-information/health-topics/weight-control/health_risks_being_overweight/Pages/health-risks-being-overweight.aspx#k.

National Institutes of Health, National Library of Medicine. Medline Plus. 2015. "Iodine in Diet." www.nlm.nih.gov/medlineplus/ency/article/002421.htm.

———. "Morning Sickness." 2016. www.nlm.nih.gov/medlineplus/ency/article/003119.htm.

Nybo Andersen, A., et al. "Moderate Alcohol Intake During Pregnancy and Risk of Fetal Death." *International Journal of Epidemiology* 41:405–413, 2012.

Palmer, N., et al. "Impact of Obesity on Male Fertility, Sperm Function, and Molecular Composition." *Spermatogenesis* 2:253–263, 2012.

Ray, J., et al. "Greater Maternal Weight and the Ongoing Risk of Neural Tube Defects After Folic Acid Flour Fortification." *Obstetrics and Gynecology* 105:261–265, 2005.

Rubio-Tapia, A. "The Prevalence of Celiac Disease in the United States." *American Journal of Gastroenterology* 107(10):1538–1544, 2012.

Schmidt, R., et al. "Maternal Periconceptual Folic Acid Intake and Risk of Autism Spectrum Disorders and Developmental Delay in the CHARGE (CHildhood Autism Risks from Genetics and Environment) Case-Control Study." *American Journal of Clinical Nutrition* 96:80–89, 2012.

Schmidt, R., et al. "Prenatal Vitamins, One-Carbon Metabolism Gene Variants and Risk for Autism." *Epidemiology* 22:476–485, 2011.

Scholl, T. "Iron Status During Pregnancy: Setting the Stage for Mother and Infant." *American Journal of Clinical Nutrition* 81:1218S–1222S, 2005.

Sekhavat, L., and Moein, M. "The Effect of Male Body Mass Index on Sperm Parameters." *Aging Male* 13:155–158, 2010.

Sermondade, N., et al. "BMI in Relation to Sperm Count: An Updated Systematic Review and Collaborative Meta-Analysis." *Human Reproduction Update* 19:221–231, 2013.

Siu, A., and the US Preventive Services Task Force (USPSTF). "Screening for Depression in Adults: US Preventive Services Task Force Recommendation Statement." *Journal of the American Medical Association* 315:380–387, 2016.

Tobias, D., et al. "Physical Activity Before and During Pregnancy and Risk of Gestational Diabetes Mellitus, A Meta-Analysis." *Diabetes Care* 34:223–229, 2011.

US Department of Agriculture and US Department of Health and Human Services. *2015–2020 Dietary Guidelines for Americans,* 8th ed. "Caffeine." http://health.gov/dietaryguidelines/2015/guidelines/chapter-1/a-closer-look-inside-healthy-eating-patterns/#callout-caffeine.

———. "Shifts Needed to Align with Healthy Eating Patterns." http://health.gov/dietaryguidelines/2015/guidelines/chapter-2/a-closer-look-at-current-intakes-and-recommended-shifts/.

US Department of Health and Human Services. "Fetal Alcohol Spectrum Disorders." https://report.nih.gov/nihfactsheets/ViewFactSheet.aspx?csid=27.

———. "Prenatal Care Fact Sheet." 2012. www.womenshealth.gov/publications/our-publications/fact-sheet/prenatal-care.html#c.

US Department of Health and Human Services, Office on Women's Health. "Polycystic Ovary Syndrome Fact Sheet." 2016. www.womenshealth.gov/publications/our-publications/fact-sheet/polycystic-ovary-syndrome.html#b.

Vahratian, A., et al. "Multivitamin Use and the Risk of Preterm Birth." *American Journal of Epidemiology* 160:886–892, 2004.

Waller, D., et al. "Prepregnancy Obesity as a Risk Factor for Structural Birth Defects." *Archives of Pediatric and Adolescent Medicine* 161:745–750, 2007.

Wang, J. "Body Mass and Probability of Pregnancy During Assisted Reproduction Treatment: Retrospective Study." *British Medical Journal* 321:1320–1321, 2000.

Wong, W., et al. "Effects of Folic Acid and Zinc Sulfate on Male Factor Subfertility: A Double-Blind, Randomized, Placebo-Controlled Trial." *Fertility and Sterility* 77:491–498, 2002.

2. GREAT EXPECTATIONS: HOW EATING HEALTHY FOOD IS GOOD FOR YOU AND YOUR BABY

Academy of Nutrition and Dietetics. "Position of the Academy of Nutrition and Dietetics: Nutrition and Lifestyle for a Healthy Pregnancy Outcome." *Journal of the Academy of Nutrition and Dietetics* 114:1099–1103, 2014.

American Academy of Pediatrics. *Pediatric Nutrition Handbook*, 7th ed. Elk Grove Village, IL: AAP, 2013.

American Academy of Pediatrics, Committee on Drugs. "The Transfer of Drugs and Other Chemicals into Human Milk." *Pediatrics* 108:776–789, 2001.

American Academy of Pediatrics, Committee on Fetus and Newborn. "Controversies Concerning Vitamin K and the Newborn." *Pediatrics* 112:191–192, 2003.

American College of Obstetricians and Gynecologists, Committee on Obstetric Practice. "Moderate Caffeine Consumption During Pregnancy." 2010. www.acog.org/Resources-And-Publications/Committee-Opinions/Committee-on-Obstetric-Practice/Moderate-Caffeine-Consumption-During-Pregnancy.

———. "Vitamin D: Screening and Supplementation During Pregnancy." 2015. www.acog.org/Resources-And-Publications/Committee-Opinions/Committee-on-Obstetric-Practice/Vitamin-D-Screening-and-Supplementation-During-Pregnancy.

American Thyroid Association, Public Health Committee. "Iodine Supplementation for Pregnancy and Lactation—United States and Canada: Recommendations of the American Thyroid Association." *Thyroid* 16:949–951, 2006.

Bergmann, R., et al. "Supplementation with 200 mg/day Docosahexaenoic Acid from Mid-Pregnancy Through Lactation Improves the Docosahexaenoic Acid Status of Mothers with a Habitually Low Fish Intake and of Their Infants." *Annals of Nutrition and Metabolism Journal* 52:157–166, 2008.

Berry, R. J., et al. "Prevention of Neural Tube Defects with Folic Acid in China." *New England Journal of Medicine* 341:1485–1490, 1999.

Brenna, J., et al. "Docosahexaenoic and Arachidonic Acid Concentrations in Human Breast Milk Worldwide." *American Journal of Clinical Nutrition* 85(6):1457–1464, 2007.

Centers for Disease Control and Prevention. "Folic Acid." 2016. www.cdc.gov/ncbddd/folicacid/index.html.

Del Prado, M., et al. "Contribution of Dietary and Newly Formed Arachidonic Acid to Human Milk Lipids in Women Eating a Low-Fat Diet." *American Journal of Clinical Nutrition* 74:242–247, 2001.

Fidler, N., et al. "Docosahexaenoic Acid into Human Milk After Dietary Supplementation: A Randomized Clinical Trial." *Journal of Lipid Research* 41:1376–1383, 2000.

Food and Agriculture Organization. *FAO Fisheries and Aquaculture Report No. 978: Report of the Joint FAO/WHO Expert Consultation on the Risks and Benefits of Fish Consumption.* Rome, 25–29 January 2010. www.fao.org/docrep/014/ba0136e/ba0136e00.pdf.

Food and Drug Administration. "Final Determination Regarding Partially Hydrogenated

Oils." *Federal Register*. 2015. www.federalregister.gov/articles/2015/06/17/2015-14883/
final-determination-regarding-partially-hydrogenated-oil.

————. "Is Stevia an 'FDA Approved' Sweetener?" 2016. http://www.fda.gov/aboutfda/
transparency/basics/ucm214864.htm

Hernandez-Diaz, S., et al. "Folic Acid Antagonists During Pregnancy and the Risk of
Birth Defects." *New England Journal of Medicine* 343:1608–1614, 2000.

Innis, S., et al. "Essential Omega-3 Fatty Acids in Pregnant Women and Early Visual
Acuity Maturation in Term Infants." *American Journal of Clinical Nutrition* 87:548–557,
2008.

Jack, B., et al. "The Clinical Content of Preconception Care: An Overview and Preparation of This Supplement." *American Journal of Obstetrics and Gynecology* 199:S266–
S279, 2008.

Mayo Clinic. "Drugs and Supplements: Isotretinoin (Oral Route)." 2015. www.mayoc-
linic.org/drugs-supplements/isotretinoin-oral-route/description/drg-20068178.

National Academies of Science, Institute of Medicine, Food and Nutrition Board.
Dietary Reference Intakes for Calcium, Phosphorus, Magnesium, Vitamin D, and Fluoride.
Washington, DC: National Academies Press, 1997.

————. *Dietary Reference Intakes for Energy, Carbohydrate, Fiber, Fat, Fatty Acids, Cholesterol, Protein, and Amino Acids.* Washington, DC: National Academies Press, 2002.

————. *Dietary Reference Intakes for Thiamin, Riboflavin, Niacin, Vitamin B6, Folate,
Vitamin B12, Pantothenic Acid, Biotin, and Choline.* Washington, DC: National Academies Press, 2000.

————. *Dietary Reference Intakes for Vitamin A, Vitamin K, Arsenic, Boron, Chromium,
Copper, Iodine, Iron, Manganese, Molybdenum, Nickel, Silicon, Vanadium, and Zinc.*
Washington, DC: National Academies Press, 2001.

————. *Dietary Reference Intakes for Vitamin C, Vitamin E, Selenium, and Carotenoids.*
Washington, DC: National Academies Press, 2000.

————. *Dietary Reference Intakes for Water, Potassium, Sodium, Chloride, and Sulfate.*
Washington, DC: National Academies Press, 2004.

National Institutes of Health, National Library of Medicine. Medline Plus. "Iodine in
Diet." 2015. www.nlm.nih.gov/medlineplus/ency/article/002421.htm.

————. "Morning Sickness." 2016. www.nlm.nih.gov/medlineplus/ency/article/003119.
htm.

National Institutes of Health, Office of Dietary Supplements. "Calcium Fact Sheet
for Health Professionals." 2016. https://ods.od.nih.gov/factsheets/Calcium-HealthPro-
fessional/

————. "Iodine Fact Sheet for Health Professionals." 2011. https://ods.od.nih.gov/fact-
sheets/Iodine-HealthProfessional/.

————. "Magnesium Fact Sheet for Health Professionals." 2016. https://ods.od.nih.gov/factsheets/Magnesium-HealthProfessional/.

————. "Vitamin A Fact Sheet for Health Professionals." 2016. https://ods.od.nih.gov/factsheets/VitaminA-HealthProfessional/.

————. "Vitamin C Fact Sheet for Health Professionals." 2016. https://ods.od.nih.gov/factsheets/VitaminC-HealthProfessional/.

————. "Vitamin D Fact Sheet for Health Professionals." 2016. https://ods.od.nih.gov/factsheets/VitaminD-HealthProfessional/.

————. "Vitamin E Fact Sheet for Health Professionals." 2016. https://ods.od.nih.gov/factsheets/VitaminE-HealthProfessional/.

————. "Vitamin K Fact Sheet for Health Professionals." 2016. https://ods.od.nih.gov/factsheets/VitaminK-HealthProfessional/.

Pena-Rosas, J., et al. "Daily Oral Iron Supplementation During Pregnancy." *Cochrane Database of Systematic Reviews* 12:CD004736, 2012.

Ralston, N., et al. "Selenium Health Benefit Values: Updated Criteria for Mercury Risk Assessments." *Biological Trace Element Research.* 2016. Accessed at http://link.springer.com/article/10.1007%2Fs12011-015-0516-z.

Rothman, K., et al. "Teratogenicity of High Vitamin A Intake." *New England Journal of Medicine* 33:1369–1373, 1995.

Shaw, G., et al. "Periconceptional Dietary Intake of Choline and Betaine and Neural Tube Defects in Offspring." *American Journal of Epidemiology* 160:102–109, 2004.

Siega-Riz, A., et al. "Second Trimester Folate Status and Preterm Birth." *American Journal of Obstetrics and Gynecology* 191:1851–1857, 2004.

Sylvetsky, A., et al. "Nonnutritive Sweeteners in Breast Milk." *Journal of Toxicology and Environmental Health.* 78:1029–1032, 2015.

US Department of Agriculture, Agricultural Research Service. "National Nutrient Database for Standard Reference." www.ars.usda.gov/main/site_main.htm?modecode=80-40-05-25.

————. "USDA Database for the Choline Content of Common Foods." 2014. http://naldc.nal.usda.gov/download/47335/PDF.

US Department of Agriculture and US Department of Health and Human Services. *2015–2020 Dietary Guidelines for Americans,* 8th ed. "Appendix 12: Food Sources of Vitamin D." 2015. http://health.gov/dietaryguidelines/2015/guidelines/appendix-12/.

————. "Appendix 13: Food Sources of Dietary Fiber." 2015. http://health.gov/dietaryguidelines/2015/guidelines/appendix-13/.

————. "Chapter One. Key Elements of Healthy Eating Patterns." 2015. http://health.gov/dietaryguidelines/2015/guidelines/chapter-1/a-closer-look-inside-healthy-eating-patterns/.

US Department of Health and Human Services, Office on Women's Health. "Folic Acid Fact Sheet." http://www.womenshealth.gov/publications/our-publications/fact-sheet/folic-acid.html.

Wang, G., et al. "Association Between Maternal Prepregnancy Body Mass Index and Plasma Folate Concentrations with Child Metabolic Health." *Journal of the American Medical Association Pediatrics.* Published online June 13, 2016. doi:10.1001/jamapediatrics.2016.0845.

Zeisel, S. "Nutritional Importance of Choline for Brain Development." *Journal of the American College of Nutrition* 23:621S–626S, 2004.

3. MYPLATE PLANS: WHAT TO EAT BEFORE, DURING, AND AFTER PREGNANCY

Academy of Nutrition and Dietetics. "Position of the Academy of Nutrition and Dietetics: Nutrition and Lifestyle for a Healthy Pregnancy Outcome." *Journal of the Academy of Nutrition and Dietetics* 114:1099–1103, 2014.

American College of Obstetricians and Gynecologists, Committee on Obstetric Practice. "Committee Opinion: Physical Activity and Exercise During Pregnancy and the Post-partum Period." 2015. www.acog.org/Resources-And Publications/Committee-Opinions/Committee-on-Obstetric Practice/Physical-Activity-and-Exercise-During-Pregnancy-and-the Postpartum-Period.

Centers for Disease Control and Prevention, Division of Nutrition, Physical Activity, and Obesity. "Healthy Pregnant or Postpartum Women." 2015. www.cdc.gov/physicalactivity/basics/pregnancy/index.htm.

National Academies of Science, Institute of Medicine, Food and Nutrition Board. *Dietary Reference Intakes for Energy, Carbohydrate, Fiber, Fat, Fatty Acids, Cholesterol, Protein, and Amino Acids.* Washington, DC: National Academies Press, 2002.

US Department of Agriculture, Center for Nutrition Policy and Promotion. www.choosemyplate.gov.

———. "MyPlate Daily Checklist." www.choosemyplate.gov/MyPlate-Daily-Checklist.

US Department of Agriculture and US Department of Health and Human Services. *2015–2020 Dietary Guidelines for Americans,* 8th ed. "Appendix 2: Estimated Calorie Needs per Day, by Age, Sex, and Physical Activity Level." 2015. http://health.gov/dietaryguidelines/2015/guidelines/appendix-2/.

———. "Dietary Fats: The Basics." 2015. http://health.gov/dietaryguidelines/2015/guidelines/chapter-1/a-closer-look-inside-healthy-eating-patterns/#callout-dietaryfats.

4. YOUR PREGNANCY: EXPECT THE BEST

Academy of Nutrition and Dietetics. "Position of the Academy of Nutrition and Dietetics: Nutrition and Lifestyle for a Healthy Pregnancy Outcome." *Journal of the Academy of Nutrition and Dietetics* 114:1099–1103, 2014.

————. "Position of the Academy of Nutrition and Dietetics: Promoting and Supporting Breastfeeding." *Journal of the Academy of Nutrition and Dietetics* 115:444–449, 2015.

American Academy of Allergy, Asthma & Immunology. "Prevention of Allergies and Asthma in Children." www.aaaai.org/conditions-and-treatments/library/at-a-glance/prevention-of-allergies-and-asthma-in-children.aspx.

American Academy of Pediatrics. "Breastfeeding and the Use of Human Milk: Policy Statement." *Pediatrics* 129:496, 2012.

American Academy of Pediatrics and American College of Obstetricians and Gynecologists. *Guidelines for Perinatal Care,* 6th ed. Elk Grove, IL: AAP and ACOG, 2008.

American College of Obstetricians and Gynecologists, Committee on Obstetric Practice. "Committee Opinion: Physical Activity and Exercise During Pregnancy and the Postpartum Period." 2015. www.acog.org/Resources-And-Publications/Committee-Opinions/Committee-on-Obstetric-Practice/Physical-Activity-and-Exercise-During-Pregnancy-and-the-Postpartum-Period.

American College of Obstetricians and Gynecologists. "Repeated Miscarriage: ACOG Education Pamphlet FAQ100." 2016. http://www.acog.org/Patients/FAQs/Repeated-Miscarriages.

Artal, R., et al. "A Lifestyle Intervention of Weight-Gain Restriction: Diet and Exercise in Obese Women with Gestational Diabetes." *Applied Physiology in Nutrition and Metabolism* 32:596–601, 2007.

Buck Louis, G., et al. "Lifestyle and Pregnancy Loss in a Contemporary Cohort of Women Recruited Before Conception: The LIFE Study." *Fertility and Sterility* 106:180–188, 2016.

Centers for Disease Control and Prevention. "Diseases and Conditions: When Should a Mother Avoid Breastfeeding?" 2015. www.cdc.gov/breastfeeding/disease/index.htm.

Centers for Disease Control and Prevention, Division of Nutrition, Physical Activity, and Obesity. "Healthy Pregnant or Postpartum Women." 2015. www.cdc.gov/physicalactivity/basics/pregnancy/index.htm.

De La Rochebrochard, E., and Thonneau, P. "Paternal Age and Maternal Age Are Risk Factors for Miscarriage: Results of a Multicentre European Study." *Human Reproduction* 17:1649–1656, 2002.

Greer, F., et al. "Effects of Early Nutritional Interventions on the Development of Atopic Disease in Infants and Children: The Role of Maternal Dietary Restriction, Breastfeeding, Timing of Introduction of Complementary Foods, and Hydrolyzed Formulas." *Pediatrics* 1:183–191, 2008.

Kiel, D., et al. "Gestational Weight Gain and Pregnancy Outcomes in Obese Women: How Much Is Enough?" *Obstetrics and Gynecology* 110:752–758, 2007.

Kris-Etheron, P., and Innis, S. "Position of the American Dietetic Association and

Dietitians of Canada: Dietary Fatty Acids." *Journal of the American Dietetic Association* 107:1599–1611, 2007.

March of Dimes. "Miscarriage." 2012. www.marchofdimes.org/complications/miscarriage.aspx.

Mayo Clinic. *Guide to a Healthy Pregnancy.* Boston, MA: Da Capo Press, 2011.

National Academies of Science, Institute of Medicine. *Weight Gain During Pregnancy: Reexamining the Guidelines.* Washington, DC: National Academies Press, 2009.

National Academies of Science, Institute of Medicine, Food and Nutrition Board. *Dietary Reference Intakes for Energy, Carbohydrate, Fiber, Fat, Fatty Acids, Cholesterol, Protein, and Amino Acids.* Washington, DC: National Academies Press, 2002.

————. *Dietary Reference Intakes for Vitamin A, Vitamin K, Arsenic, Boron, Chromium, Copper, Iodine, Iron, Manganese, Molybdenum, Nickel, Silicon, Vanadium, and Zinc.* Washington, DC: National Academies Press, 2001.

National Institutes of Health, National Library of Medicine. Medline Plus. "Fetal Development." 2015. www.nlm.nih.gov/medlineplus/ency/article/002398.htm.

————. "Fetus (12 Weeks Old)." 2015. www.nlm.nih.gov/medlineplus/ency/imagepages/9572.htm.

————. "Miscarriage." www.nlm.nih.gov/medlineplus/miscarriage.html.

National Institute of Allergy and Infectious Disease. "2017 Addendum Guidelines for the Prevention of Peanut Allergy in the United States." www.niaid.nih.gov/diseases-conditions/guidelines-clinicians-and-patients-food-allergy

National Institute of Child Health and Human Development. "What Causes Pregnancy Loss/Miscarriage?" 2013. www.nichd.nih.gov/health/topics/pregnancyloss/conditioninfo/Pages/causes.aspx.

Scholl, T. "Iron Status During Pregnancy: Setting the Stage for Mother and Infant." *American Journal of Clinical Nutrition* 81:1218S–1222S, 2005.

5. THE FOURTH TRIMESTER: AFTER THE BABY ARRIVES

Ainsworth, B., et al. "Compendium of Physical Activities: An Update of Activity Codes and MET Intensities." *Medicine & Science in Sports and Exercise* 32:S498–504, 2000.

American Academy of Pediatrics. "Colic Relief Tips for Parents." 2015. www.healthychildren.org/English/ages-stages/baby/crying-Colic/Pages/Colic.aspx.

————. "Breastfeeding and the Use of Human Milk: Policy Statement." *Pediatrics* 129:496, 2012.

————. *Pediatric Nutrition Handbook,* 6th ed. Elk Grove Village, IL: AAP, 2008.

American College of Obstetricians and Gynecologists, Committee on Obstetric Practice. "Committee Opinion: Physical Activity and Exercise During Pregnancy and the Postpartum Period." 2015. www.acog.org/Resources-And-Publications/

Committee-Opinions/Committee-on-Obstetric-Practice/Physical-Activity-and-Exercise-During-Pregnancy-and-the-Postpartum-Period.

March of Dimes. "Keeping Breast Milk Safe and Healthy." www.marchofdimes.org/baby/keeping-breast-milk-safe-and-healthy.aspx.

National Institutes of Health, National Library of Medicine. Medline Plus. "Colic and Crying: Self-Care." 2015. www.nlm.nih.gov/medlineplus/ency/patientinstructions/000753.htm.

National Institute of Mental Health. "Postpartum Depression Facts." www.nimh.nih.gov/health/publications/postpartum-depression-facts/index.shtml.

Quinn, T., and Carey, G. "Does Exercise Intensify or Diet Influence Lactic Acid Accumulation in Breast Milk?" *Medicine and Science in Sports and Exercise* 31:105–110, 1999.

Wagner, C., and Greer, F. "Prevention of Rickets and Vitamin D Deficiency in Infants, Children, and Adolescents." *Pediatrics* 122:1142–1152, 2008.

Zhang, M., et al. "Study on the Effect of Moderate Exercise on Lactic Acid Content in Breast Milk by Indirect CE with Amperometric Detection." *Chromatographia* 74:275–280, 2011.

6. FOOD SAFETY BASICS: BEFORE, DURING, AND AFTER PREGNANCY

Centers for Disease Control and Prevention. "About Lead in Drinking Water." 2015. www.cdc.gov/nceh/lead/leadinwater/.

———. "At-Risk Populations." 2015. www.cdc.gov/nceh/lead/tips/pregnant.htm.

———. "E. Coli (Escherichia coli)." 2016. www.cdc.gov/ecoli/index.html.

———. "Parasites: Toxoplasmosis (Toxoplasma Infection): Frequently Asked Questions (FAQs)." 2013. www.cdc.gov/parasites/toxoplasmosis/gen_info/faqs.html.

———. "Vital Signs: Listeria Illnesses, Deaths, and Outbreaks: United States, 2009–2011." *MMWR Morbidity and Mortality Weekly Report.* 62(22):448–452, 2013.

———. "What Is Salmonellosis?" 2016. www.cdc.gov/salmonella/general/index.html.

Environmental Protection Agency. "Your Drinking Water." www.epa.gov/your-drinking-water.

———. "Basic Information About Lead in Drinking Water." 2016. www.epa.gov/your-drinking-water/basic-information-about-lead-drinking-water.

Food and Agriculture Organization. *FAO Fisheries and Aquaculture Report No. 978: Report of the Joint FAO/WHO Expert Consultation on the Risks and Benefits of Fish Consumption.* Rome, 25–29 January 2010. www.fao.org/docrep/014/ba0136e/ba0136e00.pdf.

Food and Drug Administration. "Food Safety for Pregnant Women." 2016. www.fda.gov/Food/FoodborneIllnessContaminants/PeopleAtRisk/ucm312704.htm#safe_temps.

————. "For Consumers: Keep Listeria Out of Your Kitchen." 2015. www.fda.gov/ForConsumers/ConsumerUpdates/ucm274114.htm.

————. "Pesticide Monitoring Program 2008." 2015. www.fda.gov/food/foodborneill-nesscontaminants/pesticides/ucm228867.htm#Figure_1.

————. "Safe Minimum Cooking Temperatures." 2016. www.foodsafety.gov/keep/charts/mintemp.html.

National Institute of Environmental Health Sciences. "Endocrine Disruptors." www.niehs.nih.gov/health/materials/endocrine_disruptors_508.pdf.

Ralston, N., et al. "Selenium Health Benefit Values: Updated Criteria for Mercury Risk Assessments." *Biological Trace Element Research*. 2016. Accessed at http://link.springer.com/article/10.1007%2Fs12011-015-0516-z.

US Department of Agriculture, Agriculture Marketing Service. "Labeling Organic Products." www.ams.usda.gov/sites/default/files/media/Labeling%20Organic%20Products.pdf.

US Department of Agriculture and US Department of Health and Human Services. *2015–2020 Dietary Guidelines for Americans*, 8th ed. 2015. http://health.gov/dietaryguide-lines/2015/guidelines/.

World Health Organization. "Dioxins and Their Effects on Human Health." 2014. www.who.int/mediacentre/factsheets/fs225/en/.

7. COMMON CONCERNS AND SPECIAL SITUATIONS

Academy of Nutrition and Dietetics. "Position of the Academy of Nutrition and Dietetics: Nutrition and Lifestyle for a Healthy Pregnancy Outcome." *Journal of the Academy of Nutrition and Dietetics* 114:1099–1103, 2014.

American College of Gastroenterology. "Pregnancy in Gastrointestinal Disorders." 2011. http://gi.org/wp-content/uploads/2011/07/institute-PregnancyMonograph.pdf.

American College of Obstetricians and Gynecologists. "Preeclampsia and High Blood Pressure During Pregnancy." 2014. www.acog.org/~/media/For%20Patients/faq034.pdf.

Centers for Disease Control and Prevention, National Center for Health Statistics. "Mean Age of Mothers Is on the Rise: United States, 2000–2014." 2016. www.cdc.gov/nchs/data/databriefs/db232.htm.

————. "National Prematurity Awareness Month." 2015. www.cdc.gov/features/prema-turebirth/index.html.

————. "Prevalence Estimates of Gestational Diabetes Mellitus in the United States, Pregnancy Risk Assessment Monitoring System (PRAMS), 2007–2010." 2014. www.cdc.gov/pcd/issues/2014/13_0415.htm.

Goodnight, W., and Newman, R. "Optimal Nutrition for Improved Twin Pregnancy Outcome." *Obstetrics and Gynecology* 114:1121–1134, 2009.

Heinrichs, L. "Linking Olfaction with Nausea and Vomiting of Pregnancy, Recurrent Abortion, Hyperemesis Gravidarum, and Migraine Headache." *American Journal of Obstetrics & Gynecology* 186:S215–S219, 2002.

March of Dimes. "Multiples: Twins, Triplets, and Beyond." 2015. www.marchofdimes. org/pregnancy/multiples-twins-triplets-and-beyond.aspx#.

———. "Preterm Labor and Premature Birth." 2016. www.marchofdimes.org/complications/preterm-labor-and-premature-birth.aspx#.

Mayo Clinic. "Diseases and Conditions: Gestational Diabetes." 2014. www.mayoclinic. org/diseases-conditions/gestational-diabetes/basics/complications/con-20014854.

———. "Healthy Lifestyle: Getting Pregnant." 2014. www.mayoclinic.org/healthy-lifestyle/getting-pregnant/in-depth/pregnancy/art-20045756?pg=2.

National Center for Biotechnology Information, National Library of Medicine. "Pregnancy and Birth: Weight Gain in Pregnancy." 2014. www.ncbi.nlm.nih.gov/pubmedhealth/PMH0072759/.

National Institute of Child Health and Human Development. "Preeclampsia and Eclampsia: Condition Information." 2013. www.nichd.nih.gov/health/topics/preeclampsia/conditioninfo/Pages/default.aspx.

National Institute of Diabetes and Digestive and Kidney Disorders. "Constipation." 2015. https://www.niddk.nih.gov/health-information/health-topics/digestive-diseases/constipation/Pages/all-content.aspx

National Institutes of Health, National Library of Medicine. Medline Plus. "Hyperemesis Gravidarum." 2015. www.nlm.nih.gov/medlineplus/ency/article/001499.htm.

———. "Morning Sickness." 2016. www.nlm.nih.gov/medlineplus/ency/article/003119.htm.

O'Brien, K., et al. "Calcium Absorption Is Significantly Higher in Adolescents During Pregnancy than in the Early Postpartum Period." *American Journal of Clinical Nutrition* 78:1188–1193, 2003.

Resources

GENERAL

Academy of Nutrition and Dietetics
www.eatright.org

American Academy of Family Physicians, FamilyDoctor.org
familydoctor.org/familydoctor/en/pregnancy-newborns.html

American Academy of Nurse Practitioners
www.aanp.org

American Congress of Obstetricians and Gynecologists
www.acog.org/Patients

American Gynecological Obstetrics Society
www.agosonline.org/resources.html

American Physical Therapy Association
www.apta.org

Association of Women's Health, Obstetric, and Neonatal Nurses
www.awhonn.org

Canadian Women's Health Network
www.cwhn.ca

Centers for Disease Control and Prevention
www.cdc.gov/pregnancy/during.html

Dietary Guidelines for Americans 2015–2020
health.gov/dietaryguidelines/2015/guidelines/

Dietitians of Canada
www.dietitians.ca

March of Dimes
www.marchofdimes.org

National Association of Anorexia Nervosa and Associated Disorders
www.anad.org

National Birth Defects Prevention Network
www.nbdpn.org

National Domestic Violence Hotline
www.ndvh.org

National Eating Disorders Organization
www.nationaleatingdisorders.org

National Institute of Child Health and Development
www.nichd.nih.gov

Preeclampsia Foundation
www.preeclampsia.org

Society for Maternal-Fetal Medicine
www.smfm.org

Special Supplement Program for Women, Infants and Children (WIC)
www.fns.usda.gov/wic/women-infants-and-children-wic

Office of Research on Women's Health
http://orwh.od.nih.gov

BREASTFEEDING AND POSTPARTUM

Academy of Certified Childbirth Educators
www.acbe.com

American College of Nurse-Midwives
www.ourmomentoftruth.com

International Childbirth Education Association
www.icea.org

International Lactation Consultant Association
www.ilca.org

La Leche League, International
www.llli.org

Postpartum Support International
www.postpartum.net

Sidelines High-Risk Pregnancy Support
www.sidelines.org

FOOD SAFETY

Center for Food Safety and Nutrition, Food and Drug Administration
www.fda.gov/Food/default.htm

Centers for Disease Control and Prevention
www.cdc.gov/foodsafety/index.html

Environmental Protection Agency, Your Drinking Water
www.epa.gov/your-drinking-water

National Lead Information Center
www.epa.gov/lead

Partnership for Food Safety Education
www.fightbac.org

INFERTILITY

American Society of Reproductive Medicine
www.asrm.org

Resolve, The National Infertility Association
www.resolve.org

MIDWIVES AND DOULAS

American College of Nurse-Midwives
www.midwife.org

Doulas of North America (DONA)
www.dona.org

Midwives Alliance of North America
www.mana.org

MULTIPLE BIRTHS

Multiples of America
www.multiplesofamerica.org

Raising Multiples
www.mostonline.org

ADDITIONAL READING

Exercising Through Your Pregnancy, by James F. Clapp, MD and Catherine Cram, MS. Addicus Books, 2012.

Gluten-Free Diet: The Definitive Resource Guide, 5th ed., by Shelley Case, RD. Case Nutrition Consulting, 2016.

Heading Home with Your Newborn: From Birth to Reality, by Laura Jana, MD, and Jennifer Shu, MD. American Academy of Pediatrics, 2015.

Take Two Crackers and Call Me in the Morning: A Real-Life Guide for Surviving Morning Sickness, by Miriam Erick, MS, RD. Amazon Digital Services LLC, 2015.

New Mother's Guide to Breastfeeding, by Joan Younger Meek, MD. American Academy of Pediatrics, Bantam Books, 2011.

Nursing Mother, Working Mother, by Kathleen Huggins and Gale Pryor. Harvard Common Press, 2007.

The Nursing Mother's Companion, 7th ed., by Kathleen Huggins. Harvard Common Press, 2015.

When You're Expecting Twins, Triplets or Quads: Proven Guidelines for a Healthy Multiple Pregnancy, 4th ed., by Dr. Barbara Luke, MPH, RD, and Tamara Eberlein. William Morrow Paperbacks, 2017.

The PCOS Diet Plan: A Natural Approach to Health for Women with Polycystic Ovary Syndrome, by Hillary Wright, MEd, RD. Ten Speed Press, 2017.

Index

CPSIA information can be obtained
at www.ICGtesting.com
Printed in the USA
BVOW06*1146160317
478680BV00008B/48/P